Autoimmune Disease Anti-Inflammatory Diet

30 Healthy Anti-Inflammatory Recipes to Eat Well Every Day and Improve Health Fast Without Feeling on a Diet

Alexander Great

Table of Contents

Chapter 5: Healthy Desserts and Recipes to Satisfy Your Sweet Cravings

Chapter 1: Introduction

The Benefits of the Anti-Inflammatory Diet

There are many diets and new ways of eating, including complete lifestyle changes that result in major transformations. Many diets focus on weight loss, though there are a growing trend and interest in tailoring your food choice to improve health while preventing disease and chronic conditions. Inflammation is a symptom of recurring chronic health conditions, though it is also an important way that the body heals itself during an injury or viral infection. When inflammation is constant, it can become a serious problem that can cause pain and discomfort. Changing your diet and lifestyle is easier and more satisfying than you think, and can make a major positive impact in your life for the long-term.

What are the benefits of an anti-inflammatory diet? As you change the way you eat to combat inflammation, you'll notice many other advantages occur at the same time, and many of these are beneficial to your health and wellbeing, as follows:

Reduction of Refined Sugar and Syrup

Refined and added sugars and syrups are in many of the foods we eat, including many processed and boxed cereals, baking kits, and other packaged foods that may appear to be whole and natural, though often with hidden ingredients. Once you begin switching processed foods for whole foods such as fresh fruits, vegetables, meats, nuts, dairy, and seeds, you'll notice a major impact on your health and the way you feel. Naturally occurring sugars in fruit and vegetables, for example, is a part of a balanced diet, though adding more than needed will spike blood glucose levels and contribute to excessive weight gain, heart disease, and high blood pressure. By reducing the amount of unnatural (and natural) sugars you eat by simply skipping unhealthy foods, you'll be eradicating many other health risks and conditions you may already have or want to prevent, along with reducing inflammation.

Weight Loss is Quick and Consistent

With the introduction and increase of anti-inflammatory foods, you'll notice less bloating and weight loss, both of which are common when inflammation is lessened over time. Eating a diet rich in fiber and antioxidants will keep your body's metabolism regular. Not only will you notice weight loss within a relatively quick time, but you'll also see the results last over time, as long as your good eating habits continue. Your body will become more efficient at using nutrients and using up any excessive fat stores so that you can maintain a healthy weight consistently.

More Nutrients, Less Disease

Anti-inflammatory foods are predominantly plant-based, which are high in vitamins and minerals naturally, which prevent disease and reduce the effects of chronic illness in your body. If you suffer from arthritis, chronic headaches, or inflammation, these will disappear completely or reduce significantly within a short period. You'll not only notice the benefits quickly, but consistently, and can enjoy life more fully without the impact of chronic pain and discomfort that often prevents many people from regular exercise or staying active.

Elevation of Mood

Eating an anti-inflammatory diet can have a powerful and positive effect on your mood. This can result in lower levels of anxiety and depression and a better sense of wellbeing overall. If you eat nutrient-rich foods regularly, the positive effects on your body will also brighten your mood and boost self-confidence as well. This will help motivate you to take on new projects and avoid putting off items or tasks you may have felt discouraged from in the past.

Thanks again for choosing this book, make sure to leave a short review on Amazon if you enjoy it, I'd really love to hear your thoughts.

Get the audiobook version of this title for free with a 30-day Audible trial

Click here if you are from the US:
https://www.audible.com/pd/B08LDY2D8M/?source_code=AUDFPWS0223189MWT-BK-ACX0-219642&ref=acx_bty_BK_ACX0_219642_rh_us

Click here if you are from the UK:
https://www.audible.co.uk/pd/B08LF1BSPS/?source_code=AUKFrDlWS02231890H6-BK-ACX0-219642&ref=acx_bty_BK_ACX0_219642_rh_uk

Click here if you are from the FR:
https://www.audible.fr/pd/B08LDZCLB5/?source_code=FRAORWS022318903B-BK-ACX0-219642&ref=acx_bty_BK_ACX0_219642_rh_fr

Click here if you are from the DE:
https://www.audible.de/pd/B08LF1GJWR/?source_code=EKAORWS0223189009-BK-ACX0-219642&ref=acx_bty_BK_ACX0_219642_rh_de

Chapter 2: The Focus on Alkaline-based Foods and Their Important Role

The Top Anti-inflammatory Foods for a Healthy Diet

Many foods combat inflammation that is recurring and can build your immune system's response to disease and chronic conditions. Many of these foods are also high in alkaline, which is beneficial for the body, which is slightly more alkalinebased on the pH scale than acidic. For this reason, it is important to include a balanced selection of food in your diet to ensure your body gets the appropriate nutrient levels according to the daily requirements. The following foods are known for their anti-inflammatory properties:

All Varieties of Berries

Berries are a good source of vitamins, fiber, and antioxidants, which prevent cancer and strengthen the immune system. Your risk of heart disease and type 2 diabetes are also reduced because berries contain a good balance of nutrients, some of which include anti-inflammatory effects on your body, which reduces disease. Studies involving the consumption of blueberries indicate a good immune response, while strawberries have shown to significantly reduce the signs of inflammation where it becomes chronic, resulting in pain relief while lowering blood pressure.

Broccoli

It's not only a favorite vegetable for many people, but it's also a highly nutritious option in many dishes, from casseroles, soups, skillet meals, or simply raw as a snack. A part of the cruciferous vegetable group, which also includes cauliflower and cabbage, broccoli is a delicious way to get many of the daily nutrients you need, including vitamins K, A, and C, and a lot of fiber. The antioxidant in broccoli, known as sulforaphane, not only fights cancer and disease but also reduces the likelihood of inflammation and swelling.

Cocoa and Dark Chocolate

If you enjoy the flavor of chocolate, the dark cocoa variety contains a high concentration of antioxidants that help keep your heart healthy and inflammation down. Enjoying a piece or two of dark chocolate, even daily, can prevent a lot of disease and health conditions, while improving your body's aging and keeping your arteries clear and healthy.

Tomatoes

High in vitamin C, lycopene, and potassium, tomatoes are an excellent source of nutrients for your body, which contributes to reducing inflammation. Studies have shown a significant level of protection against cancer and reducing excess weight, especially in women who eat tomatoes regularly. This can be increased further when tomatoes are stewed or cooked with olive oil.

Olive Oil

Extra virgin olive oil is the best option for your diet. It's a good source of monounsaturated fats and regularly used in salad dressings and many dishes of the Mediterranean diet. Olive oil should be stored in a dark bottle to retain its freshness. It's a good source of antioxidants (oleocanthal) and can decrease the effects of inflammation in the body. It is easily found in the grocery store and can be purchased online as well as natural food stores and farmers' markets.

Grapes

A good source of fiber and vitamins, which prevents and treats many disorders, from memory loss and Alzheimer's to eye diseases. This is due to anthocyanins, which prevent inflammation and many other conditions that impact your health. For this result, enjoying grapes regularly is one of the best foods for good health, along with boosting your immune system and lowering the risk of cancer.

Mushrooms

All mushrooms are excellent for good health and contain anti-inflammatory compounds. They are also high in selenium, fiber, vitamin B, and copper. Portobello, shiitake, and truffle mushrooms are all high in nutrients and can be enjoyed in a variety of ways: grilled, cooked, or raw. They are inexpensive and easy to find in most grocery stores and markets.

Seafood and Fatty Fish

Fish of all types is an important source of nutrients, such as calcium, healthy fats, and protein. Salmon, mackerel, anchovies, herring, tuna, and sardines are all recommended choices to include in your diet. A regular intake of fish improves your metabolism while preventing heart disease, kidney disease, and type 2 diabetes. Fatty acids in fish prevent cognitive decline and improve your body's ability to reduce inflammation and regulate metabolism.

Avocados

A natural source of healthy fats and fiber, avocados are a great option if you are following a vegan or plant-based diet, and/or prefer to reduce the number of carbohydrates you consume. Avocadoes are high in potassium, and magnesium too, which are vital for good bone health and reducing water retention. Adding just half an avocado a day works wonders for your health, by adding a wealth of nutrients in just one serving. They are excellent as topping in salads, sandwiches, or hamburgers.

Green Tea

Sencha and matcha green teas are popular and enjoyed widely. Matcha green tea is added to desserts, and smoothies, while sencha is enjoyed as a tea. Green tea is known for its high antioxidant level, which is higher than many fruit and vegetables. It's an important component that keeps inflammation down and helps prevent cancer and autoimmune conditions. Green tea can be included in your diet regularly, even replacing coffee as a caffeine boost in the morning. It's convenient and easy to find in most stores and can be stored for months.

Peppers

A significant source of vitamin C, peppers are one of the strongest anti-inflammation options to include in your diet. Bell peppers and chili peppers are both rich in quercetin, ferulic acid, sinapic acid, among other compounds and antioxidants that provide strong, positive effects on the immune system. As a result of improving overall health, peppers reduce the likelihood of chronic illness, which reduces inflammation.

Turmeric

A common spice added in Asian and Indian cuisine, usually mixed with other flavors and seasoning, turmeric has powerful anti-inflammatory properties. It's popular in many stews, soups, and dishes. Turmeric can also be pressed into juice and added to smoothies or prepared as a tea.

The benefits of foods high in alkaline and why they are important in the anti-inflammatory diet

When you choose a diet high in anti-inflammatory foods, this quickly translates to foods high in alkaline, which is exactly what the body needs to maintain optimal health. On the pH scale of 0 to 14, acidic levels range from 0 to just before 7, whereas alkaline foods are over 7 up to 14. Most foods hover around the center. The human body has a natural pH level of between 7.3 to 7.4, which means we are generally more alkaline and need foods at this level to maintain this balance and optimal health.Focusing on alkaline foods is easy when you follow an anti-inflammatory diet, as many of the foods that cause inflammation are acidic and should be either reduced or eliminated.

Following the pH Balanced Diet: Acidic Foods Versus Alkaline Foods

When considering which foods to increase and include more frequently in your diet, it's important which foods are more acidic versus alkaline. Some foods are close to the 7 point on the scale, which means they are neutral, neither acidic nor alkaline. Consider some of the following examples of foods and drinks and how they rank on the pH scale:

- Red meats, pickled foods, cheese, and dairy products high in sodium tend to rank moderate to high on the acidic side of the pH scale.
- Canned foods and boxes or processed food items tend to rank higher in basic than their fresh or frozen counterparts, including other fruits and vegetables. For this reason, they should be avoided as much as possible where fresh or fresh-to-frozen is available.
- Eggs, some grains, and bread are acidic, though moderately and can still be enjoyed as part of a regular diet, provided they are not consumed more than alkaline-based foods.

- Seafood, certain nuts and seeds, and nut-based butter can rank mildly or moderately acidic, though they also contain many health benefits and nutrients, which makes them an important part of your diet. Many of these foods are common for allergies, with nuts and fish is most likely, which can be avoided and replaced with many other plant-based alternatives that provide many of the same nutrients, such as avocado, berries, and specific seeds.
- In the neutral category, most forms of water are neither acidic nor alkaline, which includes tap distilled and spring water. Depending on the region and the possibility of pollutants, some types of water can become more acidic and harmful as a result. On the other hand, some water bottling companies promote alkaline-based water products with the claim that their water helps establish a pH balance in the body.
- Most fruits and vegetables are alkaline based, including foods that appear acidic, such as citrus fruits. Once lemons, limes, oranges, grapefruits, and other varieties of citrus fruits are consumed, they become alkaline-based in the body. Vegetables are also alkaline-based, as long as they are consumed in fresh or frozen form, without any additives or preservatives, which can alter the taste and pH level.
- Dates, avocados, melons, and green beans are examples of vegetables and fruits that tend to have a higher alkaline level on average. If you consume more acidic foods than expected,

adding a good portion of these options is a good way to balance your pH and bring your body back to a healthier level.

- Dark greens, leafy vegetables, including kale, seaweed, broccoli, and many other green (especially dark green) vegetables are ranked as the highest in alkaline and are best to include in your diet as often as possible. Lemons are considered high in alkaline as well, which may seem unlikely due to their acidic taste.

Foods high in alkaline are also anti-inflammatory and can make a major impact on your diet. Making the shift to more alkaline-based foods coincides with choosing foods that are less likely to cause inflammation in the body. Some of the commonalities associated with these goods are as follows:

- Both alkaline-rich and anti-inflammatory foods tend to be plant-based. The more plant-based foods you choose, the more you'll reduce inflammation and achieve greater pH balance in your diet. This is especially important if you have recurring health conditions associated with one or both factors, such as consuming too many acidic foods and/or eating too many foods that inflame the body.
- Choosing natural over-processed foods is always the best option for optimal health. This means avoiding smoked foods (even plant-based options), as well as canned foods and chemically dried fruits. Any changes made to natural foods will likely increase the acidic

levels and therefore impact your health. Making the change to more natural or frozen (from fresh) foods is always the best option for your body.

Foods to Avoid on an Anti-inflammation Diet

Including an abundance of plant-based, healthy foods are important for a balanced diet that will reduce or eliminate inflammation, while keeping your body's pH level at its optimal level. Choosing the right foods is part of the equation, while avoiding choices that can hinder your health and progress are just as important. If you include just as many good foods as highly acidic and inflammatory foods, you'll undo all the benefits of the anti-inflammatory diet. The following foods trigger inflammation and can increase the risk of many other conditions and diseases, including chronic illness:

Refined Carbohydrates and Sugars

In small amounts, refined foods are not harmful, though they tend to sneak their way into many store-bought baked goods and bread that we enjoy regularly. For home baking recipes, you can easily replace refined sugars with raw or natural sugars and sweeteners that are better absorbed by the body and don't spike the blood glucose level as high. For low carb diets, many people use monk fruit, stevia, and/or erythritol as a healthy replacement for sugar and syrups. Maple syrup and honey will impact blood glucose, though they are better as natural options and are an excellent source of nutrients. Refined grains, bread, and pasta are also inflammatory and should be avoided as much as possible. Choose whole-grain alternatives or items with low sugar or low carbohydrates. Many bakeries and supermarkets offer healthier options to replace refined, low-nutrient baked goods, which makes grocery shopping easier.

Desserts and High Sugar Foods

In moderation, desserts are enjoyable and will not hurt health, though regularly consuming foods high in sugar will not only slow the metabolism and increase your risk of type 2 diabetes, you'll notice higher instances of bloating, weight gain, and inflammation. There are easy and delicious ways to recreate some of your favorite desserts and treats, without the need for sugar or highly refined ingredients. This includes replacing dairy ingredients with plant-based, adding nuts and seeds to provide a good source of protein, fiber, and healthy fats, so that you can enjoy a treat guilt-free and without the concern about gaining excess weight or suffering from the effects of inflammation.

Processed Meats, Cheese, and Snacks

All processed foods, even if they are healthy and full of nutrients in their original state, should be avoided when they are processed, as they become high amounts of sodium, preservatives, and other artificial ingredients that elevate blood pressure, add toxins into the body and increase inflammation. When choosing meat and cheese products, avoid foods that are smoked or high in sodium, selecting baked, grilled, raw, or frozen. If you tend to eat these foods on occasion, make sure you drink plenty of water to flush out the sodium and increase the amount of detoxification. Snacks such as chips, pretzels, popcorn, and other salty snacks, including meat or sausage sticks, candies, and foods high in sugar and artificial coloring, should also increase blood pressure, glucose levels, and weight gain. Choose dried fruits (sun-dried instead of chemically dried), raw or lightly roasted almonds, seeds, nuts, and raw fruits and vegetables as snacks. Hummus, vegetable-based dips, and natural yogurt (both dairy and non-dairy) are ideal for snacking while maintaining a healthy, balanced diet.

Trans Fats and Processed Oils

Many vegetable oils are processed and contain trans fats, which are also found in deep-fried foods and snacks, including French fries, onion rings, burgers, and meats. Trans fats are responsible for increasing the risk of cancer, heart disease, and other conditions, including weight gain, premature gaining, and worsening the effects of chronic illness such as arthritis. Choose natural oils in their original state for salad dressings, cooking, and baking, such as olive oil, avocado oil, and coconut oil. These oils are better sources of healthy fats and do not contain the chemicals and dangerous effects that trans fats cause. As an alternative to deep-frying, baking is a better option to reduce or eliminate trans fats.

Excessive Alcohol Consumption

Drinking too much alcohol, too often, can have many negative effects on the body. This is especially worse if drinking beverages high in both alcohol and sugar, which can have a poor effect on many bodily functions, including heart health, cognitive and memory function, and weight gain. There are also higher instances of cancer and inflammation from chronic illness when consuming too much alcohol, and too often. In moderation, a glass of wine or beer is acceptable, and won't have a negative on your health if enjoyed on occasion. The key is balance and avoiding overconsumption.

Chapter 3: Basic Recipes for Beginning the Anti-Inflammatory Diet

Preparing healthy, simple recipes for your diet is easy and does not require an expensive grocery list or specialty foods that are difficult to find in your local supermarket. The following recipes can easily be made in less than 15 minutes at any time of the day, and do not require too many ingredients.

Breakfast, Snacks, and Light Meals

Creating a healthy breakfast is easy and can be done with just a few ingredients. During the week, a busy schedule is best accommodated with a simple, no-frills recipe schedule, and a more elaborate or new recipe can be enjoyed for brunch or a late breakfast over the weekend.

Poached Eggs with Steamed Asparagus

Fresh, locally grown asparagus is recommended, though if you have frozen asparagus or a handful of spinach or arugula, this will work just as well! It's important to maximize the number of dark greens you have in your diet to reduce inflammation while increasing iron, protein, and calcium. These vegetables are also high in antioxidants and fiber, both of which are vital for good health and maintaining a balanced weight.

Ingredients:

- 2 eggs (large or medium in size)
- ½ bunch of asparagus (about 6-8 spears, cut into 3-inch pieces or longer if desired)
- Dash of sea salt
- Black pepper, coarsely ground, 1 teaspoon
- Butter (1 tablespoon), optional

Directions:

1. Two medium-sized cooking pots are needed for this recipe.
2. Fill one pot with 2 cups of water and bring to a boil, with a dash of sea salt.
3. Add in the asparagus spears as the water increases to a boiling temperature, then reduce to low and cover until the vegetables soften.
4. In the second cooking pot, fill will 3 cups of water and sea salt, and bring to a boil. Break open one egg at a time and drop into the water to poach and cook until soft or hard (depending on your preference).
5. As the eggs cook, drain the asparagus and transfer to a plate, adding a light coating of sea salt and slab of butter.
6. Top with the poached eggs and lightly sprinkle ground black pepper and more salt, if desired.

Additional toppings to consider: a light sprinkle of paprika and/or parmesan cheese (dried or fresh shavings).

Tofu Scramble

A plant-based diet is a certain way of achieving a low inflammation diet while improving the level of dietary fiber and vitamins. Soy-based foods are inexpensive and an excellent way to ensure you have enough protein, calcium, and fiber in your diet, without the high-fat content of red meats and dairy. Tofu is a versatile food that can be used to create smoothies, desserts, and puddings in soft form, or bakes, salad toppings, and/or skillet meals in firm or extra firm form. It is easily located in the produce aisle or section of the grocery store. Tofu is excellent for marinating and can be spiced or flavored for any meal.

In this recipe, tofu is marinated the night before (overnight), in vegetable broth and turmeric, along with a light coating of sea salt and black pepper. Other spices can be added as preferred, such as oregano, paprika, basil, and/or chili pepper.

Ingredients:

- 1 block of tofu (extra firm)
- 3 cups of vegetable broth
- 1 teaspoon of turmeric
- 1 teaspoon of chili pepper (optional)
- ½ teaspoon of sea salt
- Basil leaves (dried, crushed)
- Paprika, ½ teaspoon
- Oregano, ½ teaspoon
- 2 cloves of crushed garlic

- 1 tablespoon of crushed onion
- Olive oil (for cooking)

Directions:

1. Rinse and drain the block of extra firm tofu and slice into 1-inch cubes.
2. Place into a medium or large container.
3. In a small or medium bowl, stir the vegetable broth with the turmeric, black pepper, and sea salt.
4. Add the other spices and mix well, then pour over the sliced tofu and cover the container with a lid to refrigerate for a minimum of two hours, or preferably, overnight. When the tofu is well marinated, drain and retain at least ½ cup of the liquid, and heat a skillet with the olive oil and toss in the crushed garlic and onions to saute on medium heat, until translucent.
5. In a medium bowl, mash the drained tofu and, if desired, add extra spice and seasoning. Toss the mashed tofu into the skillet and saute with the onions and garlic on medium. The texture and appearance will resemble scrambled eggs, due to the turmeric's yellow color and other spices added to the tofu.

Continue to cook the tofu for 3-5 minutes, or until a bit darker in color, then serve in a bowl or plate topped with your choice of fresh chopped parsley or green onions. For a boost of fiber, add a few fresh slices of fruit to the side to enjoy. If not all the tofu is enjoyed, it can be refrigerated and reheated within the next 2 days.

Oatmeal with Apples and Cinnamon

Hot oatmeal is a great way to get the nutrients you need in the morning and can last for hours after a meal. Oats and whole grains are excellent for satisfying hunger, even in small or moderate portions, and can be enjoyed at any time of the day, though they are usually added as a breakfast food or in a food supplement. If you have gluten allergies or sensitivities, there are gluten-free oats and other whole grains without this wheat protein. Apples and cinnamon are added to this recipe to enhance the flavor and richness of this meal.

Ingredients:

- 1 cup of raw, steel rolled oats (organic is recommended; gluten-free or regular can be used)
- 2 small or 1 medium apple, sliced, cored and skin removed
- 2 tablespoons of maple syrup or raw sugar (honey or a low carb sweetener can also be used)
- 2 teaspoons of ground cinnamon
- 2 cups of water
- Dash of sea salt

Directions:

1. Pour the water into a medium cooking pot and bring to a boil with a dash of sea salt. Add in the oats and lower the heat to medium-low.

2. Toss in the sliced apples and stir in the sweetener, followed by the cinnamon.
3. If using granulated raw sugar, you may combine the sugar and cinnamon before stirring into the oats.
4. Continue to cook until the oats are done, and apples are softened, then serve topped with additional sweetener and/or cinnamon.
5. Raw brown or golden sugar is another topping to consider.
6. Serve with a dollop of coconut cream or almond milk.

Skillet Breakfast

Making a hearty breakfast can be as easy as using the leftovers from yesterday's roast chicken of tofu skillet meal. The best part of reheating or incorporating a dinner into breakfast? The ingredients are already marinated and ready to enjoy.

Ingredients:

- 3 eggs
- 3 cups of cooked or skillet-fried vegetables
- Black pepper
- Whole grain toast
- Olive oil, for cooking

Directions:

1. Heat a large skillet on medium setting or temperature with olive oil.
2. In a small bowl, whisk 3 eggs with a fork and toss into the skillet, scrambling them with a spatula.
3. Once the eggs are nearly cooked, add in the leftover skillet foods and mix well.
4. Sprinkle with black pepper, then serve with whole-grain toast.

Eggs Poached in Tomato Sauce

If you want a different taste for your morning breakfast, this is an ideal option for a late morning brunch or a simple way to use leftover tomato sauce from a previous meal or marinade. This is an easy dish to assemble and can be prepared within 15 minutes. A wide cooking pot or frying pan is recommended. If you use a single serving cast iron frying pan or skillet dish, you can serve directly. Some many spices and flavors can be added to this recipe, or you may keep it simple and minimize the seasoning for easier preparation.

Ingredients:

- Tomato sauce (or crushed tomatoes), 2 cups
- 2 eggs
- Cumin seeds, 1 teaspoon
- ½ onion, diced finely
- 2 cloves of garlic, crushed
- Olive oil, for cooking
- Sea salt and black pepper, to taste

Optional ingredients:
- 2-3 tablespoons of parmesan cheese (dried or finely grated)
- ¼ cup of shredded or crumbled feta cheese
- Chili powder, 1 teaspoon

Directions:

1. To prepare the skillet, add the olive oil and heat on medium.
2. Toss in the cumin seeds, crushed garlic and onions and saute for 2 minutes or until fragrant.
3. Add in any additional spices, such as chili pepper and/or oregano, paprika, etc., and saute for a few extra minutes.
4. Pour in the crushed tomatoes or tomato sauce. If you prefer a few chunks of tomatoes or an overall thick or chunky sauce, this can work well, as long as there is enough to cover the skillet.
5. Smooth tomato sauce can be mixed with diced tomatoes as well.
6. Once the sauce is poured into the skillet, stir with a spoon or spatula for about 3 minutes, then crack one egg into the sauce, followed by the second egg keeping them at least 2 inches apart, but also not too close to the edge of the pan.
7. Cook on medium until the eggs are firm or ready as per your preference.
8. As the eggs cook, add salt, pepper, paprika, parmesan cheese, and/or any other toppings as desired.
9. Feta cheese crumbles are best to add just before serving, as well as any chopped parsley, dill, or cilantro if desired.
10. Serve or enjoy from the skillet or scoop the contents of the pan onto a plate.
11. This dish can be enjoyed on its own or with whole-grain toast.

Spinach Omelette

This is an easy omelet that takes only a few minutes to create. Frozen, defrosted spinach works best, though fresh and fine chopped or diced works well. Other vegetables and spices can be added to enhance the flavor, and these are included in the recipe below.

Ingredients

- 3 eggs
- 2 cups of fresh spinach or 1 cup dethawed (cooked, frozen)
- Sea salt
- Paprika
- Black pepper
- Olive oil
- 2 cloves of crushed garlic
- ½ red onion, diced finely

Directions:

1. Heat a skillet on medium and add the olive oil.
2. Toss in the onion and garlic, then saute for 2 minutes until softened.
3. In a medium bowl, whisk the eggs well and mix in the minced spinach with the black pepper, salt, and other spices.

4. Pour over the fried onions and garlic on the skillet and cook for about 2-3 minutes until an omelet is formed.
5. Gently fold half of the omelet over, then flip to cook the opposite side for the same length of time.
6. Serve with whole-grain toast and/or a cup of fresh fruit.

Recipes with Five or Fewer Ingredients

If you are often too busy to prepare a meal, creating smoothies or snacks in advance can be an ideal way to satisfy your hunger, while getting the best nutrients you need daily. These recipes are quick and easy to make and can be stored for longer periods, making them available throughout a busy work week.

Avocado and Oat Milk Smoothie

Oat milk is growing in popularity, along with soy, almond, and coconut milk. It is highly nutritious and can serve to replace dairy milk in many recipes, including smoothies and as a flavor for coffee, tea, and iced drinks. If you are allergic to oats, you can easily replace and make this smoothie with almond or coconut milk, both of which are delicious and combine well with avocados.

Ingredients:

- 1 ripe avocado (soft, and slightly mushy)
- 2 cups of oat milk (or another non-dairy milk)
- 2 tablespoons of maple syrup, honey, or low carb (natural) sweetener
- 1 tablespoon of coconut cream (optional)

Directions:

1. Slice and pit the avocado, and add into the blender with the oat milk, sweetener, and coconut cream.

2. Blend for about 45-60 seconds and serve once the contents are smooth.
3. If the smoothie is too thick, add a bit more milk.
4. Serve over ice or add one or two ice cubes to crush into the smoothie, before enjoying this drink.

Banana and Avocado Smoothie

If you enjoy the taste of avocado, you may want to try this variation of the above recipe with the addition of bananas and coconut milk, which create a thicker texture and flavor twist.

Ingredients:

- 1 banana (ripe or overripe)
- 1 avocado (ripe and mushy)
- 3 cups of coconut milk (almond or oat milk can be used instead)
- 2 tablespoons of maple syrup, honey, or low carb (natural) sweetener

Directions:

1. Slice the banana and avocado and add a little at a time with the coconut milk into the blender, and pulse, adding a few slices of avocado, then banana, alternating between both until they are all combined and smoothly mixed with the milk.
2. Add in the sweetener and mix thoroughly, then serve over ice or blend (crush) ice into the drink before serving.

Mixed Berries Smoothie

All berries contain a high level of antioxidants that are ideal for the prevention of inflammation while providing a high level of vitamin C and fiber to your diet. Consuming berries on a regular diet is a great way to increase your dietary fiber while getting a good portion of your daily nutrients without the need for supplements. Just a handful of berries (the size of your palm) once each day can make a significant improvement in your diet and vitamin intake. To make your daily dose of berries interesting, you can blend them, or choose from one or more at a time: cherries, raspberries, strawberries, blueberries, blackberries, as well as gooseberries and currants, both of which may not be as widely used, and a bit sour, though make an excellent blend with sweeter berries, such as blueberries and raspberries.

Berries in this smoothie can be used frozen or fresh. If you harvest berries, they are best to use soon after collecting and rinsing them, as their flavor will remain strong and tasty.

Ingredients:

- 1 cup of berries (mixed or your choice of one or more together)
- 2 cups of milk (dairy, coconut, almond, soy, or oat milk)
- 2 teaspoons of honey, maple syrup or raw sugar (or low carb sweetener)
- ½ banana (optional)

Directions:

1. Combine the berries and pour into a blender, along with your choice of milk and sweetener.
2. Blend for about 30-40 seconds, until smooth.
3. If you want to thicken this drink, add the ½ or a whole banana, and continue to blend, or add more berries to pulse for a few more seconds.

Banana and Peach Smoothie

Peaches and bananas are naturally smooth and blend well on their own in smoothies, and often without the need for added milk. A bit of water or naturally squeezed juice is a great alternative to milk (dairy or non-dairy) if you have this available. If you choose to add milk, blend the banana with milk first, then add in the peaches to combine into the smoothie. If you are using juice in place of milk, avoid store-bought juice cartons or pre-made juice drinks, as they often contain added sugar and artificial flavors and ingredients. Juicing your drink may take some time if you have a few oranges or grapefruits to work with, or you may choose to press carrots, apples, and/or mangos into an electric juicer, if available. Some cafes or natural food stores offer fresh press juices made to order, which can be kept in the refrigerator for up to 3 days and used for a variety of smoothies or enjoyed on their own.

Ingredients:

- 2 cups of milk (any variety) or freshly squeezed juice
- 1 banana
- 1 small or medium peach (sliced, pitted and skin removed)

Directions:

1. Add the milk or juice into the blender, along with the banana and pulse for about 30-45 seconds.

2. If the mixture is too thick, add another ¼ to ½ cup of juice or milk, then pulse for another 10-15 seconds, and add in the sliced peach to thicken and blend until smooth.
3. Serve over ice or add in a few ice cubes to crush into the drink.

Peaches are best used when in season, as they will be naturally softer and easier to blend without effort into your smoothie. If unavailable, or not soft enough to use in your drink, consider fresh mangoes (small, orange mangoes work best for smoothies, due to their squishy and smooth texture), papaya, or pineapple.

Almond Butter and Chocolate Smoothie

This smoothie is ideal for getting your chocolate fix while adding a significant portion of protein, calcium, and healthy fat into your diet by blending almond butter. Almonds are highly nutritious and contain many nutrients, such as healthy fats, protein, vitamins, calcium, and fiber. Including 10-12 raw or lightly roasted almonds daily can make a major impact on the quality of your diet and health. Almond butter is a great option for smoothies because it combines an easy texture with your favorite milk to create a tasty meal replacement smoothie that can be enjoyed for breakfast or as a way to enjoy a meal when there isn't enough time.

If almond butter isn't readily available, peanut butter is a good substitute, provided it is sugar-free, low in sodium, and without any artificial ingredients. Smooth peanut butter is preferred for smoothies, as it will blend better with the other ingredients. Tahini butter, cashew nut butter, hazelnut butter, and other nut-based butter are also excellent to use, as they all have similar textures and a high nutrient level.

Ingredients:

- ½ cup of almond butter (or another nut-based butter)
- 2 tablespoons of cocoa powder (unsweetened)
- 2 cups of almond milk (or oat milk)

- 1-2 tablespoons of raw sugar, low carb sweetener, honey, or maple syrup

Directions:

1. Pour the milk and almond butter into the blender first to pulse, for about 30-40 seconds, then add in the cocoa powder and sweetener and continue to mix for another 45-60 seconds.
2. Taste test to determine if you want to add more cocoa or sweetener, or both, then blend further and enjoy.
3. Ice cubes can be added to blend into the drink, or you can add a banana for a twist in flavor.

Tahini and Maple Smoothie

If you enjoy the flavor of maple syrup, this is an excellent way to enjoy this taste with a protein-rich nut-based butter that works well in combination with maple. If you prefer to skip on maple syrup, you can add a combination of low carb sweetener or raw sugar with a teaspoon of maple flavor extract. Tahini butter is made from sesame seeds, which are high in both protein and healthy fats. This smoothie is best made with a nut-based or dairy-free milk, such as soy, almond, or oat milk. Coconut milk can be used for a creamier texture.

Ingredients:

- ½ cup of tahini (sesame butter)
- 2 tablespoons of maple syrup (or, 2 tablespoons of another sugar or sweetener with 1 teaspoon of maple extract or flavor)
- 2 cups of oat, almond, or soy milk

Directions:

1. Combine the milk, maple syrup, or sweetener and maple extract, with the ½ cup of tahini into the blender and pulse for 45-50 seconds, or until smooth.
2. Serve over ice or crush into the drink in the blender.
3. Top with a light sprinkling of cinnamon or maple flavor drizzled on top.

4. For a thicker drink with a bit of fiber, add a banana and increase the amount of milk to 1 ½ cups.

The Antioxidant Smoothie

Combining a rich serving of foods with antioxidants in the form of a smoothie is the perfect way to combat inflammation while improving many other aspects of your health. Berries are the top option for smoothies, due to their high antioxidant level, and along with matcha green tea powder, you can amplify this effect, as green tea contains a higher content of antioxidants, while giving you a boost of energy in the process.

Ingredients:

- 1 cup of berries (any variety – raspberries or blueberries are recommended)
- 2 tablespoons of natural sweetener (low carb, honey, or maple syrup)
- 2 cups of coconut or almond milk (low-fat dairy milk can also be used)
- 2 teaspoons of matcha green tea powder

Directions:

1. Combine the milk and berries in the blender first, and pulse for about 35-45 seconds, then add in the matcha green tea powder and your choice of sweetener and continue to blend for another 60 seconds before enjoying.
2. This drink is best served over ice or with crushed ice.
3. Add half a banana (overripe) or a small, ripe avocado more nutrients and a thicker smoothie.

Yogurt Smoothies

Whether you enjoy yogurt, dairy, or avoid it completely, creating a smoothie with kefir or yogurt can be an important part of an anti-inflammatory diet. There are a few key factors to consider when choosing the yogurt for your smoothie, or deciding on whether it's an ingredient you want to include:

- Is the yogurt plain, natural, and without sugar or other added ingredients? Greek or Icelandic yogurt are the best options, as they are full-fat and contain twice the protein and calcium as their regular counterparts.
- Skip the flavored yogurt and focus on the ingredients and nutritional values for the products your buy. If there are hidden sugars, syrups, or flavors, choose another option. Plain, full-fat (if you follow a low- carb diet) or low-fat yogurt without sugar are all good options.
- If you decide to skip dairy completely, you may want to consider coconut or soy-based yogurt or kefir for your diet. As these products grow in popularity, they are becoming more common in mainstream grocery stores and markets. They contain the same type of bacterial cultures that are beneficial for gut health while giving you a plant-based alternative to the diary. They may also be easier to digest and consume for people with allergies to dairy products or with lactose intolerance.
- Yogurt and kefir can work as an excellent thickening agent for smoothies and add a

pleasant flavor as well. A couple of spoons of yogurt can easily take the place of bananas or avocado if you need to thicken a smoothie without these options available.

Meal Replacements and Snacks

If you're often on the go, then you'll benefit from having a few meal-replacement options and snacks around your home, especially if you travel often or never have time to create or prepare meals during the week. One of the best options to consider is making your snacks so that you can avoid the high cost of supermarket prices, and the unwanted, unhealthy ingredients, hidden sugars, and high sodium that often are included in many snacks.

Kale Chips

In your local supermarket or natural food store, you may have noticed kale chips as a specialty snack, often promoted as natural and healthy, though also costly and without many options. Fortunately, it is a snack that can be made easily at home with just one small batch of fresh kale, sea salt, and olive oil (or coconut oil). While kale chips are not a meal replacement, they are an excellent source of fiber and calcium that can be enjoyed as a snack. By making them at home, you can avoid many of the unwanted ingredients some varieties of this snack may include in the store, such as high sodium and artificial flavors added.

Ingredients:

- 1 bunch of kale

- 1-2 tablespoons of sea salt (or pink Himalayan salt)
- 2-3 tablespoons of olive oil (coconut oil or avocado oil can also be used)

Directions:

1. Begin preparing for making the kale chips by preheating the oven to 350 degrees, and line a baking sheet or tray with either a reusable silicone mat (or parchment paper) and lightly coat in oil.
2. Wash and remove the stems from each of the kale leaves, then slice the leaves into one or two-inch pieces.
3. Make sure they are dry with a cloth or towel before coating them lightly in oil, then placing them on the tray.
4. Lightly sprinkle sea salt over each of the chips, then bake in the oven for 8-10 minutes. The result of the chips should be crispy, but not burnt or wet.
5. This is a delicate process, as even just one minute extra can slightly burn some chips, or a bit less time can keep them raw and undercooked.
6. Depending on your oven, you may want to try a couple of small batches to "test" the outcome first.

Once the chips are ready, remove them to cool for a few minutes, then enjoy. Kale chips can be stored at room temperature in a sealed bag for up to one week.

If you want to store them longer, they can be stored in the refrigerator for 2-3 weeks. Variations on making kale chips include adding dried seasoning and spices, such as dried chili pepper powder, rosemary, parmesan cheese, and/or cumin powder. By adding one or more extra spices, you may have to bake the kale chips one minute longer, if any difference is needed at all.

Peanut Butter and Chocolate Cups

These are easy treats to create and can be kept in the freezer or refrigerator until they are ready to enjoy. There is no cooking involved, aside from melting the chocolate, and cocoa powder is added to enrich the chocolate flavor. For best results, choose smooth peanut butter without added sugar and low sodium. This recipe is prepared in three layers, and a muffin tray with silicone or paper cups is required.

Ingredients:

- 2 teaspoons of cocoa powder (unsweetened, dark cocoa)
- ½ cup of dark, unsweetened (or semi-sweet) chocolate
- 1 teaspoon of butter or coconut oil
- ½-1 cup of peanut butter (unsweetened, low sodium)
- 2 teaspoons of honey, maple syrup, and/or raw sugar (or a low carb sweetener)

Directions:

1. In a small saucepan, add the butter or coconut oil with the dark chocolate and melt on low heat.
2. Once the chocolate is evenly melted, remove from the stove and mix with cocoa powder in a small bowl, along with the natural sweetener of your choice.
3. Prepare a muffin tray with silicone or paper cups and pour ½ inch (at the most) of the

chocolate mixer into each of the cups, only using as much as half of the cocoa blend. Place the tray in the freezer to chill for 20 minutes, then remove and prepare for the next layer.

4. The first (bottom) chocolate layer should be firm, though not completely frozen. Prepare the peanut butter layer by scooping at least ½ cup (no more than 1 cup) into a small bowl and add ½ inch layer on top of the chocolate.

5. Return the tray to the freezer for another 20 minutes, then remove to top with the third and final layer of chocolate.

6. Applying the remaining melted chocolate and cocoa mix, layer over the peanut butter and place it into the freezer for another 20 minutes before serving.

These treats are high in antioxidants, healthy fats, and protein. Once they have set in the freezer (with the final, top layer setting after 20 minutes), they can be stored in the refrigerator and removed immediately before consuming. They cannot be kept at room temperature, as they will melt easily.

Date, Cocoa, and Coconut Bites

These energy bites are ideal for eating on the go and can make a great option in between meals, when you need something quick for energy, or in place of a meal. The ingredients are easy to find, and no cooking is necessary to prepare this snack. Soft, crushed dates or prunes are used to sweeten this snack, which eliminates the need to add sugar or other sweeteners. If the ingredients are a bit dry when combined, add 1 teaspoon of coconut oil (or a bit more, as needed).

Ingredients:

- ½ cup of ground dates or prunes
- 2 tablespoons of finely shredded coconut
- 2 teaspoons of cocoa powder
- 1-2 teaspoons of coconut oil
- Dash of sea salt (or pink Himalayan salt)

Directions:

1. In a small or medium bowl, use a fork to coat the ground dates or prunes with the cocoa powder.
2. If they are not ground finely, add them into the food processor to grind further, then return to the bowl.
3. Coat thoroughly in coconut oil, sea salt, and cocoa powder until the mixture can form small, 1-inch balls.
4. On a flat surface, add the shredded coconut and coat evenly.

5. Roll each of the bites onto the coconut and coat thoroughly, then place it in a container or plate (covered in plastic) and refrigerate for 30 minutes.
6. Remove to serve immediately.
7. These treats will keep at room temperature for several hours and should be stored in a small bag or container to keep them fresh.

Almond Butter Cookies

Instead of a dessert, these cookies can easily be considered an excellent source of protein and healthy fats and serve as a quick meal replacement or means of energy on short notice. Like peanut butter cookies, this recipe is easy to make, and cookies can be stored up to one week at room temperature and enjoyed at any time of the day.

Ingredients:

- 1 cup of almond butter, room temperature (softened, sugar-free)
- 2 tablespoons of raw sugar or natural sweetener (honey, maple syrup)
- 1 ½ cups of almond flour, plus ¼ cup of coconut flour
- 1 teaspoon of vanilla extract
- 1 teaspoon of baking powder
- 2 tablespoons of butter, margarine or vegan butter spread

Directions:

1. Combine the almond butter, vegan or regular butter or margarine, and vanilla extract into a medium bowl. If you choose honey or maple syrup as your sweetener, add this to the bowl and mix well.
2. Mix the flour and baking powder separately, then add into the bowl and blend with a fork until the consistency is even, and the batter is

wet, but not too sticky and difficult to work with.

3. Heat the oven to 350 degrees and lightly grease a baking tray with coconut oil or butter (a silicone mat or parchment paper can also be used).

4. Form the mixture into small, 1-inch, or 2-inch balls and assemble evenly on the tray. Using a fork, gently press down to flatten each cookie, then bake in the oven for 12-15 minutes, until cookies are a bit crisp around the edges, but remain soft in the center. Remove to cool on a wire rack for about 10-15 minutes, then enjoy.

Homemade Hummus Dip

A healthy and protein-rich chickpea dip, hummus is a popular dip that is a great option as a snack or topping on a salad. It can make an excellent spread on flatbread or toast, or simply enjoyed with fresh vegetables.

Ingredients:

- 2 cups of chickpeas, drained and rinsed (or the equivalent of one can)
- 1/8 cup of tahini (sesame butter)
- 2 tablespoons of lemon
- 2 tablespoons of olive oil
- 1 teaspoon of chili powder
- 1 teaspoon of cumin powder
- 2 cloves of crushed garlic
- 3 tablespoons of water
- Sea salt and black pepper to taste

Directions:

1. Combine the chickpeas in a blender with the olive oil, garlic, tahini, water, and lemon juice.
2. Blend the ingredients for 60 seconds, or until smooth, then add in the remaining spices to blend, then remove to serve.
3. If the hummus is too thick, add a bit more water, one teaspoon at a time, and if too thin, add a bit more tahini until the texture is at the right consistency.
4. Hummus can be stored in the refrigerator for up to one week.

Roasted Beetroot Hummus

A variation on the original hummus recipe, beetroot hummus combines the iron and fiber-rich beetroot vegetable into the dip. There are two options to prepare the beetroots: by sautéing on the stovetop or baking in the oven until the vegetable is soft and suitable for adding to the blender.

Ingredients:

- 2 cups of chickpeas, drained and rinsed (or the equivalent of one can)
- 2 medium beetroots
- 1 small onion, diced
- 1/8 cup of tahini (sesame butter)
- 2 tablespoons of lemon
- 2 tablespoons of olive oil
- 1 teaspoon of chili powder
- 1 teaspoon of cumin powder
- 2 cloves of crushed garlic
- 3 tablespoons of water
- Sea salt and black pepper to taste

Directions:

1. To prepare the beets in the skillet, chop the vegetable finely and add to a heated skillet with olive oil and diced onions.
2. Cook on medium until the onions are translucent, and beets are softened.
3. Drain the beets and onions, then remove from the stove and allow them to cool for about 15-20 minutes.

4. Blend the chickpeas, water, olive oil, lemon juice, and tahini in a food processor, then combine the remaining ingredients, including the beets and onions.
5. Pulse until smooth and creamy, then serve.
6. This hummus will keep in the refrigerator for up to one week.

Oven-Roasted Chickpeas

Chickpeas are high in both fiber and protein, and preparing them into a tasty snack is an excellent way to avoid high sodium potato chips, pretzels, and other snacks that are often flavored with artificial ingredients and contribute to a higher risk of heart disease and high cholesterol. This snack is best to enjoy on the same day, shortly after the chickpeas are roasted, as they can soften after a while.

Ingredients:

- 1 large can of chickpeas or 1 ½ cups, drained and rinsed
- Sea salt to taste
- Olive oil, to drizzle over the chickpeas (extra virgin olive oil is recommended)
- Curry powder, paprika, and if desired, chili pepper

Directions:

1. Preheat the oven to a temperature of 400 degrees and prepare a large baking tray or sheet with parchment paper or a silicone mat.
2. Drain and rinse the canned chickpeas, then pat them dry thoroughly. Add them into a sealable container and drizzle sea salt and olive oil over them, then close with a lid and gently shake to coat them.
3. Add in the curry powder, paprika, and other spices, and seasoning, and continue to toss or shake in the container to coat evenly.

4. Spread them evenly on the baking tray and add more spices if desired, or if more is needed.
5. Roast the chickpeas in the oven for about 18-20 minutes, or until they are crispy. Observe them in the oven from 15 minutes onward, to ensure they do not overcook or burn, as some ovens vary, and results can be different.
6. If they are not crispy after 20 minutes, cook for another 8-10 minutes.

Remove the chickpeas once they are done, and season more if needed, while they are warm, then cool slightly and serve in a bowl. Roasted chickpeas are best to enjoy within the same day, though they can be stored in an air-tight container and consumed within 2 days.

Chapter 4: Creating Anti-Inflammatory Diet Meals for Dinner

Practical Meal Recipes for Lunch, Dinner for Home and Other Occasions

When considering what to enjoy daily, you'll find many options are included in the anti-inflammatory diet. Consider the healthiest options available: seafood, fresh vegetables and fruits, nuts, seeds, and many natural, plant-based, and/or organically raised meats and dairy. One of the top benefits of following the anti-inflammatory diet is how versatile it is, and there is no need to focus too much on calories or carbohydrates, provided you are making sound and healthy decisions about the foods you eat. In these recipes, each meal centers around an anti-inflammatory food that "sets" the plate or meal for other great options.

Skillet Salmon with Leafy Greens

This is a simple dish that doesn't require much preparation and will satisfy your appetite well with a moderately sized portion. Salmon is best fresh or frozen, and if you choose to use a few portions from your freezer, defrost them the night before, or make sure they are fully thawed before cooking. Your choice of greens can range from spinach, asparagus, broccoli, arugula, kale, or Swiss chard. These vegetables are best prepared from fresh (or thawed from frozen) by steaming them in a medium-sized cooking pot.

Ingredients:

- 3-4 salmon fillets
- Any variety of the following greens: 2-3 cups of fresh spinach (or 1 ½ cups frozen), 2 cups of sliced broccoli florets, 2 cups of fresh arugula, Swiss chard or kale
- 2 teaspoons of olive oil
- Sea salt and black pepper
- 1 teaspoon of dried dill or parsley
- Fresh lemon juice

Directions:

1. Prepare a large skillet by heating with olive oil and on medium heat.
2. Place the salmon fillets and could thoroughly, evenly on each side.
3. Sprinkle with dill, sea salt, and black pepper.
4. To prepare the greens, they can be added in a pot of boiling water to steam or sauteed on a separate skillet with a light coating of olive oil.
5. Add a sprinkle of sea salt or black pepper.
6. Serve with the salmon on a plate and drizzle with lemon juice and parsley and/or more dried dill.
7. Additional spices and seasoning include paprika and chili pepper if desired.

**Skillet Tofu and Vegetables**

Tofu is a staple in plant-based diets, though it can be enjoyed in many dishes for anyone. It's a great anti-inflammatory food that contributes to improved metabolism and a strong serving of nutrients. The choice of vegetables is flexible, as many varieties can be included in the skillet, from snow peas, cauliflower, broccoli, bean sprouts, carrots, celery, and many other options. Low sodium soy sauce and sesame seeds enhance the flavor of the tofu, which is best marinated in advance to intensify the taste.

Ingredients:

- 1 block of extra firm tofu
- Low sodium soy sauce (2 cups for marinating, 2 tablespoons for sauteing)
- ½ cup of snow peas
- 1-2 carrots, sliced
- 1-2 celery stalks, sliced
- ½ cup of bean sprouts
- ¼ cup of finely sliced mushrooms
- ½ green pepper, sliced lengthwise
- 2 crushed garlic cloves
- 1 small onion, diced
- Olive oil for cooking
- Soy sauce for marinating and cooking (low sodium is recommended)
- Sesame seed oil and miso paste for marinating

Optional ingredients (recommended):

- Dried chilis
- Ground ginger root or powder (about 1 tablespoon)

Directions:

1. For best results, marinate the tofu is recommended. This can be done in a one-hour minimum, or overnight.
2. To create the marinade, combine ½ cup of sesame oil, 2 tablespoons of olive oil, 2 tablespoons of soy sauce (low sodium), and 2 tablespoons of miso paste in a bowl.
3. Slice the extra firm tofu and coat well in the marinade, then transfer into a container and refrigerate for at least one hour.
4. Prepare the vegetables by washing and slicing them and placing them in a large bowl beside the stove. When the tofu is ready, remove from the refrigerator.
5. Heat a large skillet on medium with olive oil and add in the tofu, pan-searing for a couple of minutes on high, then lower the temperature and add in the onion, garlic, green peppers, and soy sauce.
6. Add the ginger and chili peppers, then continue to saute for 3-4 minutes on medium. Add in the remaining vegetables, except the mushrooms and bean sprouts, which are added near the end, as they cook quickly.
7. Once all the vegetables are cooked, yet slightly crispy, toss in the sliced mushrooms and bean sprouts for another couple of minutes, then remove from heat to serve. This dish can be

served over rice or noodles, or on its own with a light coating of sliced almonds, cashews, or sesame seeds.

Spinach and Apple Salad

A tangy and delicious salad that can be enjoyed as a light meal on its own, or a side dish, spinach, and apple salad is easy to prepare and can be assembled in a matter of minutes. Raw, fresh, baby spinach leaves are recommended, along with either Granny Smith or Gala apples, though any variety is good if you prefer a different style of apple. This is an ideal dish to prepare when apples are fresh and in season. For a crunchy, crispy taste, consider using Honey Crisp apples or Cortland.

Ingredients:

- 12 ounces of baby spinach leaves
- Walnut pieces, either cut in half or coarsely chopped, 1 cup (pecans can be used in place of walnuts if desired)
- Goat cheese, crumbled, ½ cup
- Large apples, 2, cut and cored, skin can be left on or peeled
- Red onion, half, peeled and sliced thinly
- Apple cider vinaigrette (one serving)
- Dried cranberries, ½ cup (raisins or another dried berry can be used if cranberries are not available.

Recipe for making apple cider vinaigrette:

- Dash of sea salt and black pepper
- Dijon mustard, 1 tablespoon
- Olive oil (extra virgin recommended), 1/3 cup
- Lemon juice, 2 tablespoons

- Apple cider vinegar, ¼ cup
- Honey or maple syrup, 1 tablespoon (low carb or an alternative sweetener can be used)
- 1 clove of garlic, shredded or crushed

To create the vinaigrette, pour all the ingredients into a bowl and whisk until well combined. Pour into a glass jar or sealable container, then shake to mix again. Set aside or in the refrigerator until ready to use.

Directions:

1. Combine the spinach leaves with the red onions, walnuts, apples, dried cranberries, and mix well in a large bowl.
2. Toss in the crumbled goat cheese and drizzle the apple cider vinaigrette on top before serving.
3. Add more goat cheese, walnuts and/or pecans if desired.
4. Sliced or slivered almonds (raw or lightly toasted) can also be added as a topping.

Eggplant Parmesan

A delicious meal that can be enjoyed on its own or with a salad or side, eggplant parmesan is not only easy to make but inexpensive and effortless to find all the ingredients needed for a tasty meal. Large or medium-sized eggplant is recommended, as it slices well and can be easily coated with the breading. This dish is baked in the oven and served with marinara or tomato sauce.

Ingredients:

- 3 eggplant (3 medium or 2 large), thinly sliced – skin can be left on or off
- 2 eggs, slightly beaten
- Breadcrumbs, 4 cups (Italian or whole-grain breadcrumbs are recommended; if following a low carb diet, use the same quantity in almond flour)
- Spaghetti sauce or tomato sauce, 6 cups
- Mozzarella cheese, shredded and divided (1 package or the equivalent of 16 ounces)
- Parmesan cheese, grated into ½ cup
- Dried basil, 1 teaspoon

Directions:

1. To prepare the oven, preheat to a temperature of 350 degrees.
2. Slice the eggplant into disks and coat in sea salt.
3. Set aside for 20 minutes to soften, then rinse with cold water and pat dry.

4. Coat each slice in the whisked eggs, then dip
    into the breadcrumb or almond flour, then
    place on a prepared baking sheet with a
    silicone mat or parchment paper.
5. If desired, add a dash of dried basil, sea salt
    and/or black pepper over each slice.

You can bake these slices for 10 minutes, or simply
add them to the following dish:

1. Pour spaghetti or tomato sauce into a baking
    dish to coat the bottom and place the eggplant
    slices into the sauce.
2. Layer with mozzarella, and add more layers,
    until all the eggplant is used up, and the top
    layer contains both tomato or spaghetti sauce
    and mozzarella.
3. If desired, add a sprinkling of parmesan cheese
    on the top.
4. Bake in the oven for about 35-40 minutes, or
    until golden on top, then remove to cool
    slightly, then slice and serve.
5. Serve eggplant with a side salad, soup, or
    whole-grain bread.
6. Whole grain pasta is another great option to
    consider.

Jackfruit Pulled "Pork"

If you are in search of a vegan version of pulled pork, jackfruit is an excellent option that provides the same consistency as meat, only with plant-based options. Jackfruit is most commonly found in canned form and is a highly nutritious food that can take the place of many types of meat for meals, including tuna and chicken, due to this rich texture and consistency. While this food can be bought fresh, it is much easier to work from out of the can. If you are concerned about sodium or preservatives, jackfruit can be gently rinsed and drained before using it in your next recipe.

Ingredients:

- Red onion, 1 small or ½ large, diced finely
- 4 cloves of garlic, crushed or minced
- Olive oil, 3 tablespoons
- Dry mustard powder, 1 teaspoon
- Smoked paprika, 1 tablespoon
- Cumin seeds, crushed or ground, 1 tablespoon
- ½ cup of Sriracha
- Tomato paste, 3 tablespoons
- Light brown or yellow sugar, 3 tablespoons
- ¼ cup of water
- Black pepper, freshly ground, and sea salt to taste
- 2 cans of jackfruit
- Whole-grain buns for serving pulled "pork."
- Avocado, ripe, softened to serve on the side

- Sauerkraut or kimchi, to serve
- Olive oil for cooking

Directions:

1. Prepare the oven to preheat to 350 degrees.
2. In a large skillet, preheat with olive oil on medium heat, then add in the onion and cook until softened.
3. This will take approximately 5-6 minutes.
4. Toss in the ground or crushed garlic cloves and cook for another minute or 30 seconds. Add the cumin, mustard, and paprika.
5. Saute the mixture until the spices are lightly toasted and aromatic.
6. Add in the tomato sauce and stir continuously for about 2-3 minutes.
7. As the ingredients are stirred gently and continually, add in the sriracha sauce and water, along with the golden or light brown sugar.
8. The items will simmer and add in the jackfruit to coat, cooking steadily for 4-5 minutes, or until done.
9. The sauce should have the consistency of barbecue sauce.

Serve the pulled "pork" jackfruit on whole-grain hamburger buns or bread, with a side of ripe avocado and/or sauerkraut.

Tuna Melt Sandwiches

A tasty and healthy sandwich to make, tuna melts are
excellent for a boost in energy and a good dose of
protein and calcium. Tuna also contains a good
source of healthy fats.

Ingredients:

- ¼ cup of mayonnaise (vegan or plant-based
  mayonnaise can be used)
- Lemon juice, ½ lemon or 2 teaspoons
- 2 cans of tuna
- Crushed chili peppers or flakes, ½ teaspoon
- 2 small or medium dill pickles
- Celery, finely diced, about 1 stalk
- Red onion, finely diced, about ½
- Fresh or dried parsley, 2 tablespoons (fresh is
  recommended)
- Ground black pepper and sea salt to taste
- Butter (about 1-2 teaspoons)
- 4-6 slices of bread (or as many as you need to
  make sandwiches), preferably whole grain brad
- Tomato, 1 medium or large, sliced
- Cheddar cheese or vegan cheese, sliced into 4-6
  pieces

Directions:

1. To prepare for this recipe, preheat the oven to
   400 degrees.

2. Combine the following ingredients in a large or medium bowl: lemon juice, mayonnaise, and red pepper flakes or powder.
3. Open both cans of tuna and drain any water, then add both cans to the mayonnaise and stir well.
4. Stir in the parsley, celery, pickles, red onion, and parsley and blend well.
5. Add sea salt and freshly ground black pepper.
6. Prepare each slice of bread by adding butter to each side, then add the tuna salad mixture to the opposite or unbuttered side.
7. Add a slice of tomato and one or two slices of cheese to each slice, then add the second slice of bread on top, until all sandwiches are ready.
8. Place on a baking sheet lined with parchment paper or a silicone mat and bake for about 6-8 minutes, or until cheese is melted, then serve.

Creamy Coconut Curry Pumpkin Soup

This is an aromatic and delicious dish for any diet, which contains all plant-based ingredients and can be prepared easily at home with minimal equipment. The ingredients in this dish are high in alkaline and soothing during the colder seasons or as a side dish. This soup can serve as a complete meal and provides a lot of nourishment in just one bowl. If fresh pumpkin is in season and preferred, this can be used provided all the seeds are removed from the flesh, and the inside of the pumpkin is measured accurately and blended into a puree. Using fresh pumpkin is a lot more work, and worthwhile, though using the canned option is more convenient, and there are good brands with little or no preservatives available.

Ingredients:

- Coconut oil, ¼ cup (MCT oil can also be used, if available)
- Chopped onions, 1 cup (yellow or white)
- Sea salt, ½ teaspoon
- Curry powder, 1 teaspoon
- 2 cloves of garlic, minced or crushed
- Vegetable broth, 3 cups
- Red pepper flakes, 1 teaspoon (or powder)
- Coriander, ground, ½ teaspoon
- 1 cup of coconut milk
- 1 can of pumpkin puree (or the equivalent if fresh, and in season)

Directions:

1. In a large or medium cooking pot, heat the coconut oil on a medium temperature, and stir in the garlic and onions.
2. Saute these ingredients until they are soft and translucent, which takes about 5-6 minutes.
3. Blend in the curry powder, sea salt, coriander, red pepper flakes, and vegetable broth and continue to cook.
4. Continue to cook and stir the contents of the pot until there is a slight boil, which should take about 8-10 minutes.
5. Maintaining the same temperature for cooking, cover and cook for another 18-20 minutes, and continue to stir once every couple of minutes.
6. After this time frame, reduce the heat and whisk the pumpkin puree and coconut milk to simmer and cook for another 5-6 minutes.

Once the above steps are completed, remove the cooking pot from the stove to cool for a few minutes. Pour the soup into a food processor or blender, working in small batches (no more than filling half the blender at a time) and mix until the contents are smooth. Pour back into the pot when done and reheat gently on medium before serving. Garnish with a dollop of sour cream (dairy or vegan, or coconut cream), nutmeg, and/or lightly toasted pumpkin seeds.

Miso Soup with Noodles

This is a highly nutritious soup for one major reason: it contains a miso base that is high in many nutrients, including fiber, vitamin B12, calcium, and protein. It is also a simple recipe to create and can be enjoyed alongside a main meal or as a light dish on its own. As a full meal, this soup provides a rich source of 9f vitamins and minerals for good health.

Ingredients:

- ½ cup of water
- Vegetable broth, 3 cups
- Soba noodles, about 3 ounces in total, divided in half or thirds
- Crushed red pepper or powder, ½ teaspoon
- Heated or shredder ginger, 1 tablespoon
- White or yellow miso, 1 tablespoon
- Green onion, sliced, about ½ cup
- 1 carrot, sliced or shredded
- Snow peas, whole or sliced in half, 1 cup
- Extra-firm tofu, 1 block, sliced into small cubes
- Bell pepper, sliced into small pieces
- Sriracha sauce or chili flakes (optional)

Directions:

1. Pour the vegetable broth into a large cooking pot or saucepan and add the water.
2. Bring the mixture to a boil and toss in the soba noodles, letting the noodles cook and boil continuously for about 10 minutes.

3. Cover and reduce the heat to medium and cook for another 5-6 minutes.
4. Add in the tofu cubes (drained, rinsed, and cut into cubes), along with the miso, ginger, crushed red pepper, miso paste, onions, bell pepper, and continue to cook for another 4-5 minutes.
5. Stir into the snow peas, carrots, and continue to cook until the vegetables become tender, but not overcooked.
6. Serve in bowls, and if desired, add sriracha and/or chili pepper spice for heat.

Are you enjoying this book? If so, i'd be really happy if you could leave a short review on Amazon, it means a lot to me! Thank you.

Spicy Chili with Jackfruit

Jackfruit is an amazing and versatile food that can be added as a central ingredient in many recipes. It's great for absorbing many flavors while mixing well with other plant-based ingredients and spices.

Ingredients:

- Olive oil or avocado oil, 1 tablespoon
- Carrots, ½ cup
- Celery, ½ cup
- Crushed or minced garlic cloves, 3
- Red onion, small, minced or diced finely
- Green chilies, diced 2 tablespoons
- Red pepper, 1/2cup
- 2 large cans of diced tomatoes
- Cooked kidney beans 4 cups
- Small can of tomato sauce
- 1 large can of jackfruit (in water), rinsed and drained
- Coconut or raw sugar, 1 tablespoon
- Sriracha sauce, 1 tablespoon
- Tomato paste, 1 tablespoon
- Chili powder, 2 tablespoons
- Smoked paprika, 2 teaspoons
- Cumin seeds (crushed or ground), 2 teaspoons
- Cayenne pepper, 1 teaspoon
- Dried thyme, 1 teaspoon
- Nutritional yeast, 2 tablespoons
- Liquid smoke, 2 teaspoons
- Sea salt and black pepper

- ½ lime (juice from the lime)
- 1 teaspoon of liquid aminos

Directions:

1. To prepare the jackfruit, place the can in a colander to drain and rinse.
2. Use a fork and/or spoon to mash the jackfruit into tiny pieces.
3. In a large skillet, add olive oil on medium heat and add in the garlic and onion.
4. Saute for a few minutes until the onion is softened and translucent.
5. Toss in the sliced celery, bell pepper, and carrots and continue to saute for a few minutes.
6. Add the jackfruit and green chilies and cook longer, for another 5-6 minutes, or until the jackfruit water is fully immersed in the ingredients of the skillet.

Combine the following ingredients into the skillet with the jackfruit:

1. liquid aminos, beans, tomato sauce, diced tomatoes, sriracha sauce, tomato paste, all the spices, herbs, and raw or coconut sugar.
2. Cook until contents are brought to boiling, then keep at this temperature for a few minutes, and reduce to a low- medium level of simmer for about 30 minutes.
3. Once the chili is cooked for half an hour, add the nutritional yeast, sea salt, black pepper, and liquid smoke.
4. Cook for another 5-6 minutes, then serve.

5. A bowl of chili is great with one or two slices of
    whole-grain bread or toast or a side salad.

Steamed Asparagus with Sliced Almonds and Parmesan

A side dish that works well with a baked salmon steak or roast chicken, this meal can be enjoyed as a light lunch or dinner. If parmesan cheese is not available, or you prefer to use a plant-based alternative, vegan cheese or coarsely ground cashews are another option.

Ingredients:

- 1 bunch of asparagus (if the bunch is large, use half or two thirds)
- ½ cup of raw, sliced almonds (they can be lightly toasted if desired)
- ¼ cup of fresh, grated parmesan cheese or the equivalent in vegan cheese (the same amount can be used for ground cashews)
- Sea salt
- Ground black pepper
- Butter or vegan margarine (spread)
- 3-4 cups of water

Directions:

1. In a large or medium cooking pot, bring 3-4 cups of water to a boil, adding in a dash of sea salt.
2. Slice the asparagus into 3 or 4-inch pieces, after trimming the stems, and toss into the water to cook until tender, which should take about 10-12 minutes. The asparagus should be tender, but not overcooked.

3. Drain from the cooking pot and serve on a plate or bowl.
4. Top with sliced almonds and shredded parmesan cheese (dried parmesan can be used if fresh is unavailable).
5. Sliced almonds can be lightly dry toasted for 1-2 minutes in a skillet on high heat, then cooled and topped on the asparagus; this process can be done in advance, and toasted almonds can be stored at room temperature or in the refrigerator.

Cream of Broccoli Soup

This soup recipe is known for its creamy taste and texture, though it originally includes a lot of dairies, which can be difficult for people with lactose intolerance or allergies. This recipe is different from other plant-based versions of soups that usually substitute dairy milk and other ingredients for vegan versions. In this recipe, raw cashews are used to create the base of the soup.

Ingredients:

- Olive oil, 2 teaspoons (extra virgin olive oil is recommended)
- 2 onions, medium in size, diced finely
- Carrots, 3 chopped into small disks
- Raw cashews, ¾ cup (soaked in water)
- Sea salt, 2 teaspoons
- 6 cups of water
- Ground black pepper to taste
- Broccoli, about 8 cups, sliced into small florets
- Celery, 2 stalks, chopped into small pieces
- 3 cloves of garlic, crushed

Directions:

1. To prepare the cashews, place them in a bowl (small or medium in size) and cover in water.
2. Soak overnight in a container or pour hot (boiling) water over the cashews and soak for 15-30 minutes.
3. This process will soften the nuts so they are easy to blend in a food processor. In a large

cooking pot, add the olive oil and heat on medium.

4. Add in the onion and a dash of sea salt to saute for 2-3 minutes, then combine the carrots and celery and cook for another 5-6 minutes.
5. Toss in the crushed garlic, then the broccoli and saute for longer, about an additional 6-7 minutes.
6. Once the ingredients are tender, pour in 5 cups of water, along with the sea salt and ground black pepper.
7. Continue to cook and bring all the ingredients to boiling, then reduce and simmer on low for about 16-18 minutes.

Rinse and drain the cashews and add them to one cup of water in a food processor or blender. Pulse until the mixture is creamy and smooth, with no chunks or pieces of cashews left. Place the mixture aside and puree the contents of the soup in the cooking pot in a blender or food processor. Make sure the soup has cooled for a few minutes, by removing the pot from the stove, then blend the mixture in small batches. Combine the pureed soup with the creamy cashew blend and mix well. Add a dash of sea salt, black pepper, and/or paprika to serve.

Zucchini Pasta Noodles with Shrimp and Garlic

If you enjoy garlic sauteed shrimp and zucchini noodles, this is an ideal recipe that combines these two flavors and textures into a delicious meal. Zucchini noodles, also known as "zoodles," are a low carb replacement for regular wheat-based noodles, which can contribute to inflammation. In moderation, whole grain pasta is a healthy part of a balanced diet, though it is best enjoyed in small portions with heaping servings of tomatoes, olive oil, and other foods high in fiber, vitamins, and healthy fats. Zucchini noodles can be bought in the spiral form at many grocery stores, either fresh or frozen, or you can slice or create your long noodle shapes using a circular peeler and one or two fresh zucchinis.

Ingredients:

- Olive oil, 1 tablespoon
- Shrimp, ¾ pounds or one small package, washed and peeled (small to medium shrimp work best)
- 2 medium zucchini to peel, or the equivalent already made into noodles or "zoodles."
- Fresh parsley, chopped (dried can be used, though fresh is recommended)
- Sea salt and ground black pepper to taste
- Chili or red pepper flakes (optional)
- 4 cloves of garlic, crushed
- Juice from 1 lemon, and the zest

Directions:

1. If using zucchini in the whole form, use a peeler to create the noodles, then set them aside in a bowl.
2. In a large skillet, add the olive oil and heat with the lemon juice and zest.
3. After about 2 minutes, the pan should be warm enough to add in the shrimp.
4. Cook for one minute on each side, then add in the crushed garlic cloves and red pepper (and/or chili) flakes.
5. Continue to saute for a few minutes, and frequently stir, coating the ingredients in the pan.
6. Add in the zucchini noodles and toss them evenly with a fork or tongs.
7. Repeat this process for another 3 minutes until the zoodle are lightly cooked, but not too tender or overcooked.
8. Add a dash of sea salt and ground black pepper, then toss in the chopped parsley and serve immediately.

A few optional toppings to consider include sliced toasted almonds, and/or a light dusting of parmesan or shredded vegan cheese.

Green Curry Bowl

If your taste buds are feeling adventurous, this is a mild, yet tasty dish that is not only easy to create but requires just a handful of ingredients that you may already have in your pantry. Green curry paste is common in most grocery stores and can also be found in many specialties and/or natural food stores as well (including Asian supermarkets). If you are unable to find it locally, it can be easily located and purchased online. Green curry paste, or any curry powders and/or pastes are ideal to have on hand for a variety of soups, marinades, and dishes.

Ingredients:

- 1 block of extra firm tofu
- Olive oil, a little to drizzle and a dash of sea salt
- Sweet potatoes (medium or small in size), peeled and cut into cubes
- Green curry paste, 4 tablespoons
- Broccoli florets, 3 cups
- Coconut milk, 3 cans

Ingredients for toppings (optional):

- Fresh, chopped cilantro
- Raisins (golden) or dried cranberries
- Fish sauce and/or brown sugar to sprinkle (to taste)

Directions:

1. Rinse and drain the extra firm tofu, then pat and press the tofu to remove excess water. Slice the block of tofu into cubes and set aside.
2. Add the olive oil in a soup cooking pot on medium heat, then add in the tofu, with a sprinkle of sea salt, and fry for about 12-14 minutes, or until the tofu is golden in color. Remove the cooked tofu from the pot and set aside.
3. In the same soup pot, add in the sweet potatoes, curry paste, and coconut milk.
4. Simmer on low to medium heat until the potatoes are tender and soft, then add in the broccoli and tofu.
5. Saute for another 5 minutes until the broccoli is light green.
6. Add two tablespoons of raisins, and the cilantro (if you decide to use these toppings for the recipe), then the dash of fish sauce and/or brown sugar over the top.

This curry is best served with pasta or long grain rice. If you do not prefer shrimp, salmon, chicken, or tuna can be used instead of or together in this recipe.

Salmon Patties

Fish cakes or patties are simple and fun to prepare at home, and these can be a great alternative to hamburgers and/or chicken breast for dinner. This recipe follows the Paleo diet and includes natural ingredients that are also beneficial for weight loss. Salmon patties can be refrigerated for up to one week or stored in the freezer for one month or longer. Canned salmon is most convenient to use, and there are good quality brands to choose from, though if you prefer using baked salmon, remove the skin and mash the salmon into flakes with a fork. If you have leftover baked salmon from a previous meal, this is a perfect way to use it in a new, tasty recipe for your next dish.

Ingredients:

- 3 cloves of garlic, crushed or minced
- Sweet potato or squash, mashed or pureed into 1/3 cup (pumpkin can be used instead)
- Coconut Flour, 4 tablespoons
- 1 large can of salmon, or the equivalent in baked salmon, mashed into small flakes with a fork
- 2 eggs
- Sea salt, ½ teaspoon
- Ground black pepper, ¼ teaspoon
- Smoke paprika, ½ teaspoon (or regular paprika can be used)
- Butter or olive oil, 1 tablespoon (for cooking)
- Curry powder, ¼ teaspoon

- Rosemary herb (fresh or dried), 1 teaspoon (if using fresh herbs, diced finely)

Directions:

1. To use squash in this recipe, slice the vegetable in half and remove all the seeds, then bake in the oven for about 25-30 minutes.
2. If the squash is difficult to slice in half, poke with holes (using a fork) and bake for about 15 minutes at 350 degrees in a preheated oven, then remove, cool slightly, and cut in half.
3. Return to the oven for another 20 minutes or until the inside of the squash is soft and easy to scoop out.
4. Canned squash can be used if it is not available fresh.
5. Canned, pureed pumpkin is another option, as well as fresh.
6. Sweet potato can be baked or boiled and drained before mashing, along with a dash of sea salt.
7. If you are using canned vegetables, an extra amount of coconut flour or egg white may be needed to ensure the mixture binds well.
8. 1 tablespoon of whey protein (unflavored) can be used to substitute the same amount of coconut flour in the recipe.
9. Collagen powder is another option to use to boost the protein content.
10. To begin preparing this recipe, mash the salmon into flakes (either canned or baked), removing any bones and skin attached, then place the salmon in a bowl.

11. Add the portion of mashed sweet potato, pumpkin, or squash and continue mashing the ingredients together well.
12. Add in the coconut flour and/or 1 tablespoon of whey protein or collagen and continue to mix.
13. Blend in the herbs and seasoning, and once the ingredients are well combined, add in the eggs last, then mix further until a thick batter is formed.
14. Create enough portions to make about 6-8 balls (roughly 2-3 tablespoons each), then place them on a baking tray.
15. Heat a large or medium skillet on medium heat with butter or olive oil, then press down the patties until they are about 1 inch in thickness, then place them into the heated skillet to cook on both sides for about 3-4 minutes each.
16. The patties will be well cooked once the salmon is thoroughly done.
17. Canned salmon will cook slightly faster than baked salmon.
18. Once the patties are cooked, remove them from the skillet and onto a plate to cool slightly, then add a bit more oil or butter to cook the next one or two patties.

When all the patties are cooked, serve garnished with rosemary, chili flakes or powder, garlic, and/or black pepper. To create a dip or sauce, consider making your tartar sauce by mixing ½ cup of mayonnaise (vegan mayonnaise can be used) and ½ cup of green relish. Add a bit of sriracha sauce or a dash of

cayenne pepper for extra spice. As a side dish,
steamed vegetable, a small bowl of miso soup or salad
works well.

Vegan Pizza

At first glance, many people may consider skipping a dish without any dairy or meat products, though this is a delicious meal that deserves a chance in your kitchen. To make this recipe easy, store-bought or bakery prepared pizza dough is recommended, either regular whole grain dough or gluten-free dough. There are many plant-based toppings to include, such as dried and fresh tomatoes, broccoli, basil leaves, vegan cheese and meat alternatives, black olives, and many more! For a bit of spice, consider using chili pepper or sauce drizzled on top.

Ingredients:

- 1 16-ounce package of pizza dough (available in local grocery stores or bakeries)
- Basil leaves, ½ dried or fresh
- Thyme leaves, 2 tablespoons
- Head of broccoli florets, chopped into small, bite-sized pieces, including the stalk, about 1 cup
- Cherry tomatoes, sliced in half, 1/3 cup
- 1 ear of corn, kernels removed
- Olive oil for drizzling and brushing the pizza, extra virgin oil is recommended
- Red pepper flakes to taste
- Jalapeno, ½ cup, sliced thinly
- ½ cup of sliced pitted black olives
- Red onion, sliced into chunks, about ¼ cup
- Vegan cheese (1 cup)
- Sea salt and ground black pepper

- 2 tablespoons of tomato paste

Directions:

1. Preheat the oven to 450 degrees.
2. In a large or medium bowl, combine the tomatoes, corn, onion, jalapeno pepper, dried tomatoes, and other toppings to include on the pizza.
3. Toss the vegetables in the bowl to coat them well in the olive oil and add in the seasoning to shake and coat more.
4. Set the bowl of vegetable toppings aside to work on the pizza dough.
5. Stretch the dough to knead for about 10-12 minutes, gently, then place and press into a 14-inch pizza pan.
6. Brush the edges of the dough with a light coating of olive oil and add the vegan cheese into the center of the dough, spreading it around carefully, so that it covers the dough evenly.
7. If desired, mix the tomato paste with the vegan cheese before adding to the pizza, or add the paste first, followed by the cheese (if layering the tomato paste with cheese, consider using shredded vegan cheese).
8. Distribute the vegetable toppings on the pizza evenly, then drizzle sauce and/or spices and seasonings and bake in the oven for about 15 minutes or until the crust is golden in color.
9. Broccoli should be roasted and tender. Remove from the oven and add a few more

spices and shredded cheese, as desired, then slice and serve.

Spaghetti Squash Bake

Whole wheat spaghetti noodles are not the best option for everyone, especially if you have sensitivities to wheat and/or gluten. There are gluten-free noodles and similar options available, though many products are rice or vegetable-based and may not produce the same consistency as expected. While there are some excellent products without gluten and wheat available, there is another option to recreate your favorite spaghetti dishes without using wheat at all, by using spaghetti squash. This is a delicious, nutrient-rich vegetable that contains noodle-like flesh that can be easily baked and used in many recipes and served out of the shell as well.

Ingredients:

- 1 medium or large squash, sliced in half lengthwise
- Olive oil for baking and cooking
- Vegan or dairy cheese, 2 cups, shredded (mozzarella or cheddar, or a mix)
- 1 green pepper, diced
- 1 small onion, diced
- 2 crushed garlic cloves
- Crushed chili peppers, 1 tablespoon
- Parmesan cheese (or the equivalent in vegan cheese), ¼ cup
- 2 cups of pureed or crushed tomatoes
- Ground black pepper and sea salt
- Paprika, 1 teaspoon
- Dried oregano, 1 teaspoon

- Dried or fresh basil leaves, 1 teaspoon
- ½ cup of finely sliced mushrooms

Directions:

1. In a large skillet, heat with one tablespoon of olive oil, then add in the garlic and onions to saute for a few minutes, followed by green pepper, chili peppers, and mushrooms. Cook for another 5 minutes on medium heat, then remove from the stove.
2. Slice spaghetti squash in half, then bakes in the oven for about 10-15 minutes, until softened in the center.
3. Place both halves, with the inside facing up, on a baking tray.
4. In a medium or large bowl, combine the skillet fried ingredients with tomato sauce and spices.
5. Use a fork to "pick" up and mix the spaghetti-like flesh inside each half of the squash, so that it is each to coat and mix with the tomato sauce mix, then coat each half on the tray.
6. Add a layer of vegan or dairy cheese (shredded), followed by additional spices, seasoning, and parmesan cheese.

Bake both halves of the squash on a baking sheet or tray lined with a silicone mat or parchment paper and a light sprinkle of olive oil. Preheat the oven to 375 degrees and bake for about 25-30 minutes, or until squash is tender and cheese is melted. Each half of squash can serve as a meal on its own, and be served with whole-grain toast or a side of soup or salad.

Ginger and Carrot Soup

A hearty and tasty soup, ginger, and carrot are perfect as ingredients together and provide a lot of antioxidants and vitamins in one serving. Butternut squash is used in this recipe, and it's always recommended to have at least one or two types of squash on hand, in case of a recipe. Squash comes in many different shapes and mellow flavors, which makes it an ideal ingredient to include with many of your recipes.

Ingredients:

- Olive oil, 1 tablespoon
- Carrots, chopped finely, 3 cups
- 1 leek, sliced into bite-sized pieces (green onion can be used if leek is unavailable)
- Fennel seeds or bulbs, chopped, about 1 cup
- Butternut squash, 1 cup chopped (pumpkin or more carrots can be used instead)
- Vegetable broth, 3 cups
- Sea salt and ground black pepper
- Ginger, grated, about 1 tablespoon
- Garlic cloves, minced or crushed (2)
- Turmeric powder, 1 tablespoon
- 1 can of coconut milk

Directions:

1. In a large saucepan, add the olive oil and heat at a medium temperature.

2. Add in the leeks, fennel, carrots, and squash
    together, stirring frequently, and cooking for
    about 4-5 minutes.
3. The vegetables should be softened or tender at
    this point.
4. Add in the ginger, sea salt, turmeric, garlic,
    ground black pepper, and continue to saute for
    a few more minutes.
5. Pour in the coconut milk and vegetable broth,
    and continue to stir for a few minutes, reducing
    to medium-low, then cover and simmer for
    another 20 minutes.
6. The soup should be cooked after this time
    frame.
7. Remove the soup from the stove and set aside,
    then blend in small batches until it is creamy
    and smooth, returning the batches together
    into the large saucepan or cooking pot.
8. Add seasonings and heat to serve. Serve with a
    dollop coconut cream or yogurt.

Grilled Portobello Mushrooms

A great alternative to cooking with steak, chicken, and fish, portobello mushrooms offer a wealth of nutrients in one serving and can add a delicious flavor to any dish, whether you choose to grill, saute, bake, or fry them. This is a simple recipe that works well for anyone new to cooking with portobello mushrooms. They are unique in texture and have been used as buns or patties in hamburgers, sliced and grilled as a meat replacement, or steamed for soups and skillet meals.

Ingredients:

- 3-4 portobello mushrooms
- Olive oil or avocado oil, ¼ cup
- Onions, chopped (about 3 tablespoons)
- Sea salt, ground black pepper, and seasonings of your choice
- 2 cloves of garlic, crushed or ground

Directions:

1. Clean the portobello mushrooms and remove the stems, which can be used later.
2. Heat the grills on a barbeque and wait until they are ready to grill.
3. In a small bowl, pour the olive or avocado oil, along with the crushed garlic cloves, vinegar, and crushed onions.
4. Use a brush to lightly coat each of the mushroom caps, then place each one on the grill and cook for about 10 minutes, then serve

immediately, and top with sea salt, ground black pepper, and other spices or seasoning as desired.

5. To strengthen the flavor of the mushrooms, consider soaking the caps in the oil mix for at least one hour, then grill on the barbecue to serve.

Serve the grilled portobello mushrooms with fried onion rings (these can be baked in the oven or added to the grill, as long as they are sliced thick). Baked potatoes, chili, and other sides, including a fresh salad, will work well with mushrooms to provide a complete meal.

Watermelon Salad

A refreshing dish in the summer months, watermelon salad combines the best of tangy, sweet, and savory in one meal. This dish can be enjoyed on its own or as a companion to a meal or dish at a community potluck or party. It's a popular salad that will be enjoyed in no time, and it is best to consume immediately after preparation for the best results. Aside from the ingredients in the list below, there are other options to consider as additional flavors, depending on personal taste and preference, such as green onion, green peppers (or bell peppers), and/or cucumber.

Ingredients:

- Watermelon pieces, sliced into cubes or balls, 3 cups
- Lime juice, 1 tablespoon (lemon can be used if lime is unavailable)
- Olive oil, 3 tablespoons
- Finely chopped mint, 2 tablespoons, dried or fresh leaves
- Feta cheese crumbles, 1/3 cup
- Sea salt and ground black pepper
- ½ green pepper, diced with seeds removed (optional)
- 1 ½ cups of cucumber cut into cubes with seeds removed
- Green onion, diced into small pieces

Directions:

1. In a large bowl, gently mix the watermelon, cucumber, and mint and toss evenly to blend.
2. Add any further ingredients you wish to include.
3. Mix the olive oil, lime or lemon juice, sea salt, and black pepper in a small bowl to create the dressing, then drizzle over the salad.
4. Fold in the crumbled feta and serve.

Four Ingredient Tomato Salad

This is a simple recipe that includes just four ingredients and a few options to consider for your dressing. This is a perfect summer or fall salad idea that can be served as a light snack or as a side dish. It takes only a few minutes to prepare the ingredients and serve.

Ingredients:

- 3 large tomatoes, diced into small cubes
- 1 bunch of green onion, diced into one-inch chunks (fresh leek can also be used if available)
- 1 large or 2 medium cucumbers, diced into cubes (the same size as the tomatoes)
- 2 cups of finely shredded feta or goat cheese, or feta crumbled

Directions:

1. Combine the diced cucumbers, tomatoes, and onions into a large bowl and toss evenly. Sprinkle the finely shredded feta or crumble to gently fold into the mix, or add to a single serving on top once the salad has been added to a plate or serving-size bowl.
2. No salad dressing is required, though there is the option of adding a light vinaigrette or dressing if desired.
3. To create your own, add 3 tablespoons of lime or lemon juice with a pinch of rosemary herb and 1 tablespoon of olive or avocado oil.

4. Whisk in a small bowl, then drizzle over the salad to serve, along with the shredded or crumbled feta cheese.

Cucumber Salad

A light and creamy salad, this recipe is a perfect option if you want a bit more involved in the ingredients and enjoy a creamy dressing instead of a vinaigrette. This salad includes sour cream, though yogurt (dairy or vegan) can be used as well. Some natural foods stores or grocers may offer vegan sour cream as an option.

Ingredients:

- Thinly sliced cucumbers, 3 cups (peeled and sliced)
- Sour cream, ½ cup
- Red onion, sliced thinly, 1 cup
- Fresh or dried dill, 1 tablespoon (fresh is recommended)
- Raw sugar, 1 teaspoon
- White vinegar, 1 tablespoon
- Sea salt, ½ teaspoon
- Garlic powder, ¼ teaspoon

Directions:

1. Stir in the sour cream, vinegar dill, sugar, garlic, and sea salt in a medium bowl well, then toss in the cucumbers and red onions to coat them evenly.
2. Once the ingredients are well combined, transfer to a container that can be sealed with a lid and refrigerate for 2 hours.
3. Remove from the refrigerator to serve.

4. This salad can be stored up to one week in the refrigerator.

Avocado Salad

A perfect serving of both fiber and healthy fats, this salad features avocado just before it has completely ripened. This recipe is easy to assemble and can be prepared in just a few minutes.

Ingredients:

- 2 small or 1 large avocado, slightly ripe but not too mushy
- 1 tablespoon of olive oil
- 2 tablespoons of lime or lemon juice
- Ground black pepper, ½ teaspoon
- Dash of sea salt
- 1 small tomato, diced
- ½ green pepper, diced
- ½ teaspoon of paprika

Directions:

1. In a small bowl, combine the olive oil, lemon or lime juice, and paprika.
2. Whisk together; they set aside.
3. Remove the skin and pits from the avocados and slice into cubes or strips, then add to a bowl along with the green peppers and tomato.
4. Lightly drizzle the dressing and add a dash of sea salt and ground black pepper.

Mango Salad

A sweet and tangy dish, this combines the tartness and slightly sweet taste of mangos with mint, cashews, red peppers, and spices. This is a simple variation from the traditional style of this recipe, which is popular in Thailand. Mangoes do not have to be completely ripened to include in the salad and work best if they are firm.

Ingredients:

- 1 cup of coarsely chopped cashews (they can be used in the whole form if desired)
- 2 tablespoons of dried mint leaves or freshly chopped mint
- Red pepper, sliced lengthwise into strips, one medium in size
- 2 mangos, not too ripe, skin and pits removed and sliced into strips

Directions:

1. Assemble all the ingredients into a large bowl and serve.
2. No dressing or toppings are necessary, though if you prefer the additional flavor, consider a splash of lime juice, and a dash of black pepper, freshly ground.

Choosing Nutrient-Rich Foods and Ingredients for Your Recipes

One of the most important aspects of shopping healthy and choosing the right foods for an anti-inflammation diet involves the quality of food, aside from what to eat. The source of food is just as important because the quality determines how nutritious they are, and whether they will provide enough vitamins and minerals as they are expected. For example, many grocery stores will reduce the pricing on older vegetables and fruits, which may be a good bargain at times, though if the product is improperly stored and treated, it may cause more harm than good! Reviewing the foods that you buy for good quality and where they are sourced is a vital step in making sure you get the best quality for your diet:

- Local and in-season fruits and vegetables are strongly recommended, as they are fresh and in prime condition when harvested. If they are local, this means there is less preservation needed, and the goods can be delivered directly from the farm into the market or store.
- An organic is a good option, though this label may not always live up to its promise. Organic can mean something different in various countries and regions, and for this reason, it's best to research to determine whether this option is worthwhile. If local and organic are both options, prioritize local first, organic next.
- Always consider the reputation of the brand, supplier, or farm where the foods originate

from. You may be aware of certain practices or quality that varies from one company or farm to another, which is important in understanding the value of the food and whether you trust where it comes from. If in doubt, a quick online search and some background on the company can give you peace of mind that you are choosing the right foods, or give you more information that can guide you towards a better decision.

- If you are following a budget, track price changes, and always aim for the best quality food or product within your price range. If a food item is a bit more expensive, it may be a worthwhile purchase if the quality is high, including the source of the food (locally and/or organically grown) and with good nutrient value. With financial limitations, it becomes important to prioritize the foods you need in your home and how they play an important role in your recipes and meals.

Chapter 5: Healthy Desserts and Recipes to Satisfy Your Sweet Cravings

How to Create Desserts and Treats that are Healthy and Anti-inflammatory

Satisfying your sweet or sugary cravings is not a challenge with a few ingredient changes and a healthier approach to eating well. The following recipes are ideal of creating puddings, milkshakes, and simple, yet delicious cakes that can be enjoyed guilt-free and without the worry of experiencing inflammation as a result. Many of the ingredients used in these recipes are not only anti-inflammatory, but they are also rich in nutrients and make desserts a vital part of a balanced diet.

Chia Seed Pudding

This is an excellent snack that can also be enjoyed as a dessert or for breakfast. Chia seeds are the main feature of this pudding, which helps milk or yogurt "gel" into a pudding-like texture and provide a wealth of nutrients including protein, antioxidants, calcium, fiber, and vitamins. The easiest chia seed pudding to make is vanilla, though many flavors and toppings can be added according to your preference. It's a common dish enjoyed in both the ketogenic and Paleo diets because it skips high carbs and processed foods for a natural approach to eating well. Chia seeds are easy to find in most grocery stores and can be purchased in a package or bulk. The following recipe is the easy, basic version that can be a base for many other options, including a variety of flavors and textures.

Ingredients:

- 1 ½ cups of milk (coconut milk or almond milk are recommended)
- ½ cup of cream (dairy or non-dairy, full-fat cream)
- 2 tablespoons of honey, maple syrup, or a low carb sweetener
- ¼ cup of chia seeds (any variety)
- 1 teaspoon of vanilla extract

Directions:

1. Pour the milk, cream, and vanilla extract in a large bowl.
2. Use a whisk to combine these ingredients, then add in the sweetener of your choice, followed by chia seeds, and mix well.
3. You'll notice some of the chia seeds will stick to the whisk, which is natural, and most of the seeds will mix evenly throughout.
4. Once the ingredients are well blended, pour the mixture into a bowl and cover with plastic or a sealed container, then refrigerate for a minimum of two hours, or overnight. Remove the pudding and check the consistency; it should be thick, pudding-like or gel-like in texture, and ready to enjoy!

5. If you want to include toppings, consider adding crushed nuts, fresh berries, or dried fruits as a topping.

Chocolate Chia Seed Pudding

If you enjoy the vanilla or basic chia seed pudding, you're ready to experiment with other flavors and textures that can be enjoyable and provide a good variety to your dessert menu. Because of the high nutrient value in chia seed pudding, you can enjoy these snacks as a meal replacement, or for breakfast, when you may need a good source of energy to start your day. Cocoa powder or dark chocolate can provide an additional boost to your energy along with the protein and fiber of chia seeds. You can choose a milk that is dairy or plant-based, and the sweetener you add can be raw (honey or maple syrup) or any variety of low carb options.

Ingredients:

- 1 ½ cups of coconut or almond milk (dairy milk can also be used)
- ½ cup of cream (dairy or an alternative)
- 3 tablespoons of pure, unsweetened cocoa powder (or dark melted chocolate)
- 1 teaspoon of vanilla extract (optional)
- 2 tablespoons of honey, maple syrup or a natural sweetener of your choice
- ½ cup of chia seeds

Directions:

1. If you add melted dark chocolate to this recipe, place the equivalent of 3 tablespoons into a small cooking pot or saucepan and melt on low

temperature, with one tablespoon of milk added.

2. Once the chocolate is completely melted, remove from the stove to cool for a few minutes, then stir into a bowl with the cream, milk, and vanilla extract.
3. Mix well with a whisk, then add in the sweetener.
4. If using cocoa powder, combine after mixing the wet ingredients first, then whisk in the chia seeds until they are evenly distributed throughout the blend.
5. Chill for a minimum of two hours or overnight, then serve in a bowl.
6. Top with shredded coconut, crushed nuts (peanuts, hazelnuts, or slivered almonds) or chocolate shavings or a light dusting of cocoa powder.

For a slight change in flavor with the chocolate or cocoa, consider adding a tablespoon of hazelnut butter or crushed hazelnuts. Crushed or pureed almonds are another good option to consider for a richer taste.

Pistachio Chia Seed Pudding

If you want a different twist on chia seed pudding flavor, consider adding a dose of crushed, raw (unsalted) pistachios. These nuts are strong and pleasant in flavor and often provide a delicious flavor on their own. They can be added as a topping, though infuse more flavor when they are mixed with the pudding ingredients. Pistachios are high in healthy fats and fiber.

Ingredients:

- 2 cups of coconut milk
- 2 tablespoons of cream (dairy or coconut)
- 2 tablespoons of crushed or finely ground pistachio nuts
- ½ cup of chia seeds
- 2 teaspoons of honey, maple syrup, or sweetener
- Vanilla extract, 1 teaspoon

Directions:

1. In a bowl, pour the coconut milk and cream, then whisk together with the natural sweetener.
2. Continue to stir while adding the chia seeds, then add the vanilla extract and pistachios. Once all ingredients are well combined, transfer into a container or bowl with a lid and store in the refrigerator for two hours or overnight.

3. Once the pudding is ready, remove and serve
    with additional crushed pistachios on top, or
    with a light dusting of cardamom spice.

Almond Butter Chia Pudding

Almonds are one of the best nuts to include in your diet. They are high in healthy fats, protein, calcium, and fiber. They are versatile and can be added to many types of dishes and desserts, including cookies, skillet (stir fry) meals, bakes, puddings, or as a snack on their own. Almonds are readily available in many stores and markets and are best to consume raw or lightly roasted, preferably without salt or added flavors. In this dessert, almond butter is combined with a ground meal to create a rich, textured custard combined with chia seeds for a high level of both protein and healthy fats combined. This is an ideal snack in small amounts and is ideal for increasing your energy quickly, without the need for a full meal.

Ingredients:

- ½ cup of almond butter (smooth, unsalted and unsweetened)
- 1 tablespoon of ground almond flour or meal
- 2 cups of almond or oat milk
- ½ cup of cream (dairy or coconut cream)
- 2 tablespoons of natural sweetener (honey, maple syrup or raw sugar)
- ½ cup of chia seeds
- 1 teaspoon of almond extract

Directions:

1. Combine the milk, cream, and almond extract and whisk well in a bowl.

2. Add in the sweetener, followed by the almond
   butter, almond meal, and chia seeds. Once all
   ingredients are combined, and mixed well,
   pour into a container with a lid and refrigerate
   for two hours or overnight.
3. This chia pudding is a bit thicker than other
   varieties, due to the combination of almond
   meal and butter, and may not require two full
   hours.
4. Once the pudding is ready, serve with sliced or
   slivered almonds (raw or lightly toasted) on
   top.

Vegan Sponge Cake

A simple, yet fulfilling treat to enjoy for dessert, sponge cake is often high in sugar and dairy, though this option reduces both the sugar and sticks with all plant-based ingredients. This is an ideal option for a base that can be used to add many varieties of toppings, from the jam and fresh fruit to chopped nuts, sauces, and syrups. There are many plant-based and sugar-free (or reduced sugar) options available.

Ingredients:

- Vegan margarine or coconut-based butter, ½ cup
- Almond, oat, or coconut-based milk (or another dairy-free milk), 2 cups
- Vanilla extract, 1 teaspoon
- Cider vinegar, 1 tablespoon
- Baking soda, 1 teaspoon
- Golden sugar (or low carb alternative), 1 ½ cups
- All-purpose flour, 2 cups (gluten-free flour or almond flour can be used in the same amount)

Filling:

- Sugar-free or natural marmalade or jam (raspberry or strawberry is recommended, though any flavor can be used), 4 tablespoons
- Icing sugar, 1 ½ cups, or the equivalent in honey, maple syrup or low carb (sugar-free) equivalent

- Vegan margarine or coconut-based butter, ½ cup

Directions:

1. Prepare the oven by preheating the temperature to 350 degrees and prepare two cake tins with a light coating of non-stick spray or coconut oil (vegan butter can also be used for this purpose).
2. In a small bowl or jug, combine the vinegar and non-dairy milk and whisk well.
3. Set aside for a few minutes, until this mixture becomes lumpy and frothy.
4. Add in the vanilla extract and blend further.
5. In a separate bowl, add the remaining cake ingredients and blend well.
6. Pour the milk blend over the dry ingredients and combine well, using an electric mixer or handheld blender.
7. Once the blend is ready, pour into two cake tins (dividing the batter into two equal portions), making sure an even amount is poured into each, then bake in the center rack of the oven for 30-32 minutes, or until they are ready.
8. The center of each cake should come out clean with a toothpick.

Place the cakes on a wire rack to cool and make the filling as they chill. In a small bowl, add the vegan butter or coconut-based spread and whisk with the icing sugar and jam. If you have any leftover vanilla extract or flavor, this can be added as well. Mix well with an electric blender or mixer and be careful not to overmix, as the spread may become too stiff and difficult to spread on the cake layers. Spread the mixture on the top of both sponge cakes and assemble one on top of the other. Use the leftover spread to coat the remainder of the cake or leave it just in the center (between the two cakes) and the top layer.

Decadent Brownies

This recipe is excellent for chocolate lovers and includes only plant-based ingredients, which means you'll avoid inflammation-causing foods and can simply enjoy this treat without any concerns about high sugar or unhealthy ingredients. The items included in this recipe are easy to find and can be adapted to suit a variety of dietary needs, including gluten-free flour or low carb (coconut and almond flour blend) options.

Ingredients:

- 2 cups of all-purpose flour (the equivalent can be replaced with gluten-free flour, or replace with the following blend: 1 cup almond flour, 1 cup coconut flour)
- Raw or coconut sugar, 2 cups, or replace with 1 cup of honey, maple syrup or low carb sweetener
- 1 cup of cocoa powder (unsweetened)
- Baking powder, 1 teaspoon
- Water, 1 cup
- Sea salt, 1 teaspoon
- Coconut oil or olive oil, 1 cup
- Vanilla extract, 1 teaspoon

Directions:

1. Prepare the oven by preheating to 350 degrees.
2. Combine the flour, cocoa powder, baking powder, and sea salt in a large bowl (all the dry ingredients) and stir to combine well.

3. In a separate bowl, mix the coconut oil or olive
    oil with the water and vanilla extract, then pour
    into the bowl of the flour mix and blend until
    all ingredients are well mixed. Prepare a
    baking pan with a light coating of coconut oil or
    spray, then pour the batter evenly into the pan.
4. Bake in the oven for 28-30 minutes, then
    remove to cool for 10-12 minutes. Slice into
    squares and serve.

To double the chocolate sensation of this recipe, add
½ cup of dark, semi-sweet chocolate chips to the
batter, or top the brownie batter in the tray with chips
before baking. Other options for flavor include
adding slivered or sliced almonds, chopped pecans or
walnuts, or a bit of orange or peppermint extract for a
slight twist in the flavor.

Mango Milkshake

A simple yet fulfilling treat to enjoy, this milkshake tastes more like ice cream and can be enjoyed as a summer treat in place of many high sugar and artificially flavored drinks. Fresh mangoes are recommended for this recipe, though papaya or peaches can be used instead. This milkshake can be created within just a few minutes in your blender.

Ingredients:

- 1 large or 2 medium ripe avocados
- 2 teaspoons of natural sweetener (honey, maple syrup or raw sugar)
- 2 cups of coconut milk
- 1 scoop of sugar-free ice cream (non-dairy is recommended, or skim milk)
- Dash of cardamom powder

Directions:

1. Pour the coconut milk, natural sweetener, and ice cream into a blender and pulse for about 45-50 seconds.
2. Mangoes are sliced, skins removed, and pitted before added to the blender.
3. Pulse for a few more minutes, then remove and serve with a light dusting of cardamom powder.

Other options to consider for this milkshake include:

- Adding crushed pistachios into the blender

- One extra scoop of ice cream and/or one tablespoon of plain Greek yogurt
- Adding cardamom powder into the blend (about 1 teaspoon), as well as a topping

Banana Bread Loaf

This is a recipe that traditionally includes a lot of wheat and sugar, while this recipe switches many of the inflammation-inducing ingredients for healthier options. Coconut flour and almond flour are used in place of whole wheat flour, and raw or alternatives to sugar can be easily used in place of refined sugar. This recipe is suitable for vegan and low carb diets, including Paleo. Bananas are a good source of fiber and potassium, which is important for reducing inflammation and water retention, both of which can become common and recurring with age and chronic illness. Both coconut and almond flours are mixed, as coconut flour can be a bit dry in baking, while almond can provide just the right amount of moisture for balance and good results in baking.

Ingredients:

- Coconut flour, ¼ cup
- Almond Flour, 2 cups
- Baking powder (gluten-free can be used), 2 teaspoons
- Cinnamon, 2 teaspoons
- Walnuts, ½ cup (chopped or coarsely ground)
- Butter, softened at room temperature, 6 tablespoons
- Sea salt, ¼ teaspoon
- 4 eggs, large
- Xanthan gum, ½ teaspoon (optional)
- Almond or vanilla extract, 2 teaspoons
- 2 bananas, overripe

- Almond milk, unsweetened (coconut or oat milk can be used as well)

Directions:

1. Preheat the oven to 350 degrees and lightly coat a loaf pan with olive oil or butter. Parchment paper or silicone mat can also be used, if available, followed by a light sprinkling of butter or olive oil.
2. If the parchment paper is used, make sure it hangs out the sides of the pan, so that it can be easily removed after baking the banana bread loaf.
3. In a large bowl, combine the dry ingredients, including coconut flour, almond flour, baking powder, sea salt, and cinnamon.
4. In a large bowl, mash the bananas and add in all the wet ingredients, including the almond milk, almond or vanilla extract, eggs, and other ingredients.
5. Once these items are well combined, gently pour in the dry mixture in small batches, ensuring that it blends evenly, until all the flour is mixed.
6. Continue to mix until a dough or batter forms, then stir in the walnuts and pour the batter into the prepared loaf pan.
7. If desired, leave a few chopped walnuts for the top of the loaf and sprinkle with additional cinnamon or nutmeg.
8. Bake in the oven for about 60 minutes, then use a toothpick to ensure it is done when finished.

9. If the loaf is not completely baked, return to the oven for another 10-15 minutes, then test again with the toothpick.
10. All ovens vary, and it may take a bit more or less time to fully bake the banana bread.

Cool the loaf on a wire rack completely before slicing and serving. It will slice easier if left to cool longer, though it can be enjoyed slightly warm as well. Banana bread will keep well at room temperature in a sealed container or plastic for up to 3 days, or in the refrigerator for up to one week. If planning to use at a later date, consider storing in the freezer for longer, up to a month or longer, if needed. Other options for baking banana bread include adding chopped pecans instead of walnuts or dark chocolate chips.

Pumpkin Bread Loaf

As an alternative to banana bread, pumpkin loaf is another great tasting dessert or treat that can be easily made at home, and with common ingredients. If you have a combined pumpkin spice option in your pantry, you may substitute 3 teaspoons of this mix for the nutmeg, cinnamon, allspice, and cloves below. Pureed pumpkin from the can is convenient and recommended (using the best brand with little or no preservatives), or fresh pumpkin flesh can be used to produce the same recipe. If you use fresh pumpkin, retain some of the removed seeds for a topping option.

Ingredients:

- Baking soda, 2 teaspoons
- Baking powder, 1 teaspoon
- 4 large eggs, beaten or whisked
- Ground nutmeg, 1 teaspoon
- Ground allspice, 1 teaspoon
- Ground cloves, ¼ teaspoon
- Sea salt, 2 teaspoons (finely ground)
- The ground cinnamon, 1 teaspoon
- Water, about 2/3 cup
- 1 can of pureed pumpkin (about 15 ounces)
- Unsalted butter or olive oil to grease the baking pans or loaf pans
- 2 cups of almond flour, combined with 1 ½ cups of coconut flour
- Sugar (raw or coconut sugar), 3 cups, or 2 cups of low carb sweetener

- Olive oil or coconut oil, 1 cup

Directions:

1. To prepare the oven, preheat to a temperature of 350 degrees, and use the butter or oil to lightly coat two loaf pans (9 by 5 inches), and sprinkle a light coating of flour over the top.
2. In a medium bowl, whisk the sugar and oil together, then add in the eggs and pumpkin puree and continue to whisk until well blended.
3. In a separate bowl, combine the baking soda, baking powder, sea salt, flours (coconut and almond), nutmeg, cinnamon, allspice, and cloves, and mix well.
4. Pour half of the dry ingredients into the pumpkin puree blend and stir continuously to blend.
5. Add half of the water and continue to stir to blend.
6. Continue by adding the remaining flour or dry ingredients mix, followed by the remaining water, until all ingredients are well blended.

Split the batter into two portions and pour each into a prepared loaf pan. If desired, add lightly toasted or raw pumpkin seeds on top of each loaf, then sprinkle with a dash of cinnamon or nutmeg (or pumpkin spice). Bake in the oven for about one hour, then remove to cool on a rack for about 10-15 minutes. Allow the loaf to cool completely before slicing to serve. Pumpkin bread is excellent with butter or vegan spread, or on its own. Coarsely chopped pecans and/or walnuts can be added to the batter before baking for a twist in flavor.

Chocolate Chip Cookies

An easy and fun treat to create and enjoy chocolate chip cookies can be much healthier than their store-bought counterparts. The key to making desserts and treats better in quality and nutrients lies with the quality of foods used and how nutrient-rich they are. For example, dark chocolate is the best option for recipes, as it contains antioxidants and fiber that benefit the body. The type of sweetener, flour, and whether supplements or "boosters" are added to the batter are all factored into the quality of the cookie.

Ingredients:

- 1 cup of flour (coconut and almond flour blend, ¼ cup coconut and ¾ cup almond flour), or whole-grain flour (oat or spelt flour can be used)
- Baking soda, ½ teaspoon
- Sea salt, ¼ teaspoon
- Raw sugar or coconut sugar, ¼ cup
- Brown sugar (or yellow/golden sugar), ¼ cup
- Milk, 2 tablespoons (dairy, oat, soy, almond or another option)
- Dark, semi-sweet chocolate chips (or unsweetened), 1/3 cup
- Olive or coconut oil, 2 tablespoons
- Vanilla extract, ¼ teaspoons

Directions:

1. Combine all the dry ingredients into a large bowl, including the flours, baking soda, sugars, sea salt, etc.
2. In a separate bowl, add the remaining, wet ingredients until well blended, then combine the two mixtures in one bowl.
3. A dough will form and should be even and consistent in texture.
4. Add a bit of milk if the cookie dough is too dry or not easy to work with.
5. Form into a large ball and refrigerate for two hours or freeze for about 30 minutes or until the dough is cold.
6. Just before you're ready to remove the dough from the freezer or refrigerator, preheat the oven to 325 degrees.
7. Prepare a tray with a light coating of oil or butter, then place the cookie dough in portions, with at least 1-2 inches in between.
8. Bake on the center rack of the oven for about 12-13 minutes.
9. At this stage, they may not look fully done, though they will cool and fully firm when they are removed at this time as they cool on the wire rack.
10. If there is extra cookie dough, another batch can be made at once, as the oven remains heated.
11. Alternatively, the dough can be refrigerated or frozen and used at a later date.

Zucchini Muffins

A unique and tasty batch of muffins, zucchini is a healthy and anti-inflammatory option for baking loaves and muffins. These are naturally high in fiber and vitamins and can serve as a light snack, dessert, or breakfast. Zucchini muffins can be stored at room temperature for up to 3 days, in the refrigerator for up to one week, or frozen for longer. They make an excellent fix in between meals or as a quick solution for a meal replacement. The ingredients in this recipe are common and easy to find. Gluten-free flour can be used in place of whole wheat flour, or a combination of almond and coconut flour can also be added instead.

Ingredients:

- Unpeeled zucchini, shredded, approx. 2 cups
- 1 ripe banana, mashed
- Coconut or avocado oil, ¼ cup
- Honey or maple syrup, ¼ cup
- 2 large eggs, preferably at room temperature
- The ground cinnamon, 1 teaspoon
- Vanilla extract, 1 teaspoon
- Brown or golden sugar, ¼ cup
- Baking soda, ½ teaspoon
- Baking powder, ½ teaspoon
- Sea salt or pink Himalayan salt, 1 teaspoon
- All-purpose flour (whole grain flour, spelt flour or gluten-free can be used), 2 cups
- Dark chocolate chips, 1/3 cup (semi-sweet or unsweetened)

Directions:

1. To prepare for the recipe, preheat the oven to a temperature of 375 degrees and line muffin tray with silicone or paper cups.
2. Lightly butter or grease each of the cups and set aside.
3. Use a grate to slice the zucchini into fine strips until the full vegetable is used.
4. Place the shredded zucchini on a paper towel and squeeze out as much liquid or water as possible.
5. Continue to pat dry and squeeze until there is no liquid left in the shredded zucchini, then place aside.
6. In a small saucepan, melt the coconut oil on low heat or let it soften in advance at room temperature, so that it is liquid and smooth.
7. In a large bowl, combine the banana, honey or maple syrup, brown sugar, coconut oil, and vanilla extract until it is smooth.
8. Blend in the eggs and continue to mix, making sure that the coconut oil does not become solid and remains warm or at room temperature.
9. In a separate bowl, combine the baking soda, baking powder, cinnamon, and sea salt and blend well.
10. Add in the flour and gently, gradually sprinkle and mix into the liquid mixture.
11. Use an electric mixer on low speed to make sure all the ingredients blend well, then once everything is evenly combined, fold in the shredded zucchini and chocolate chips.

12. Pour the batter into the prepared muffin cups and add a few extra chocolate chips to the top of each muffin.
13. Bake into the oven for 22-25 minutes, or until it comes out clean when a toothpick is inserted into the center of each muffin.
14. Remove the muffins from the oven and allow them to sit for a few minutes, before transferring them to the rack to cool completely.
15. Muffins can be enjoyed right away, or stored in a sealable container at room temperature for up to 3 days.
16. They can keep in the refrigerator for up to one week.

As an alternative to chocolate chips, chopped walnuts or pecans can also be folded into the batter before cooking. Shredded carrot is another optional ingredient that can be used with the zucchini or in place of it.

Chapter 6: Recreating Your Favorite Meals with Anti-inflammatory Foods

Key foods to identify as high-risk and replacing them in common recipes
The recipes included in this book are your starting point towards a healthy, balanced diet that provides many benefits, including the elimination or reduction of inflammation in the body while providing a sustainable and healthy way of eating. To further improve and enhance the balance of nutrients and quality in your diet, you may consider making easy, everyday changes to the way you eat and the foods that you choose. For some people who may have difficulty getting started on a new path of eating well, making small, yet meaningful changes can make a significant difference. Consider the following easy switches and simple habits you can implement, today for a healthier tomorrow:

Switch Refined Bread and Pasta for Whole Grain Options

Every recipe offers a healthier way towards eating better, but the simplest changes are most profound, starting with the type of food staples you purchase at the local farmer's market or grocery store. Switching your white, refined pasta noodles and bread for whole-grain options may seem a bit more expensive, though many stores offer good rates on high-quality foods. Local markets and bakeries can also provide a good price, as well as local goods room which is good for the economy and your budget! If you're not sure which whole grain products to choose, consider trying one option at a time, and ask your local bakery for recommendations on which whole grain bread is tastiest and most nutrient-packed. For pasta, flours, and other refined foods, consider researching which, while grain options are best in quality and work well within your budget. Make a point of trying one product or option at a time, to find out if it makes a good fit into your cuisine.

Replace Sugar with Fruit and Natural Alternatives

In most foods we consume, there is at least a small amount of sugar, and while this is reasonable to expect in fruits and natural foods, there are many food products with added sugars, many of which are refined and excessive. Carbonated drinks and beverages, specifically soda, as well as fruit juices and premade milkshakes, are all loaded with artificial sugar and flavors, which can spike glucose levels while increasing the risk of inflammation. Trading in high sugar sodas and drinks with unnatural sugar substitutes is easy considering the number of low carb beverages and sparkling water options available in many stores. Drinking water regularly will also ensure you are well hydrated and keep sugar levels normal in your body. Instead of buying candies and sugary treats, try naturally dried or fresh fruits as a snack.

Change High Sodium for Spices and Seasoning

There are many varieties of spices, flavors, and seasonings that can easily replace salt in many dishes and recipes. If you choose to include salt, either pink Himalayan salt or sea salt are good options because they are readily more absorbed by the body and easier to digest. Many stores offer sodium-free and low sodium options, such as soy sauce and spice blends that add a great taste or enhancement without the salt. Many store-bought foods, including snacks such as chips, nuts, pretzels, and dried vegetable chips are high in sodium, even if you can't taste it! As an alternative, consider choosing lightly roasted or raw nuts and/or seeds, and naturally dried or roasted chickpeas, zucchini, or kale chips, all of which can be made at home and for a fraction of the cost.

How to Improve the Way You Eat Today for a Healthier Tomorrow

Making changes to your diet today means you'll notice significant results over time, including in the short-term. If you find making changes difficult, you're not alone! Even the easiest diets can take time and patience to adjust to and may take a bit longer than expected. Persistence and staying consistent are two main factors that will set you on the path to success.

Chapter 7: Key Suggestions, Tips, and Frequently Asked Questions

Frequently Asked Questions

Now that you've become familiar with anti-inflammatory foods, and a collection of easy-to-follow recipes, making dietary changes will be easier and more enjoyable, especially as you discover how delicious and accessible healthy, natural, plant-based foods are and how they can be easily added into your diet while replacing processed, packaged foods commonly included in most diets.

Question: Is it recommended to follow a plant-based, vegan diet to improve the quality of diet and reduce inflammation, or is this not a requirement?

Answer: You don't have to become vegan or restrict all your foods to plant-based to enjoy a better diet, though it does help to increase the amount of plant-based foods you include, as many, if not all, reduce the incident of inflammation and improve your health overall. Red meats should be limited, though they can be enjoyed in moderation, and contain good sources of iron, protein, vitamin B12, and calcium. Controlling the amount of meat that you consume is key, and enjoying high quality (organic, free-range) options is the best way to enjoy your next serving of steak or roast.

Fish is a great option for reducing inflammation and can be included in your diet more often than other types of meat, such as poultry and red meats. If you choose to move towards a vegan or vegetable-based diet, this will make a significant impact on reducing inflammation quickly, though overall, you should be able to enjoy all types of food, in their natural form, in moderation. Keeping processed and artificially preserved foods out of your diet is the best option for good health.

Question: Is consuming too much dairy a problem for inflammation and related health problems?

Answer: In short, some dairy can be problematic, though there are good options to consider for a healthy, anti-inflammation diet. Yogurt and kefir, both fermented dairy foods, are excellent for promoting gut health and balancing the natural bacterial in your body. Plant-based versions of yogurt and kefir can also be found in some natural food stores, and a growing number of supermarkets are offering coconut milk and soy-based options as well. Cheese, milk, butter, and cream should be limited and used in moderation and small amounts. Always choose organic, natural options for dairy because the quality makes a significant difference. Avoid flavored milk and cheese, as they often have sugar or high levels of sodium. Yogurt and kefir should also be consumed plain; you can add your own choice of fruit, natural sweeteners, and toppings, all of which will not have the same level of sugar as store-bought flavored dairy foods.

Wherever possible, choose the best brands of dairy products, and opt for some plant-based alternatives, even if just to try them – you'll be pleasantly surprised how many delicious nut-based and soy-based beverages and dairy products taste. They are also excellent as milk replacements in recipes and can be used without concern about high calories and fat. Like dairy, however, some vegan milk products and dairy alternatives can contain preservatives and added sugars, which makes reading the labels and nutrient lists on each carton or container important, to make sure you're getting exactly what you want and need for a healthy diet.

Question: Are eggs acceptable to enjoy regularly on an anti-inflammatory diet, or should they be limited?

Answer: In small amounts and doses, eggs are acceptable, and can provide a great deal of support for a healthy diet, including one that decreases inflammation. Like many foods, it's important to not overeat anything, including eggs, though they are beneficial if you enjoy one or two each day, or as an ingredient in a recipe. If you choose to follow a plant-based diet or want to reduce eggs in your diet, you can replace one egg with ground flaxseeds and water (about 2 tablespoons) for your next recipe. Tofu scramble, and other soy or vegetable-based meals are excellent for replacing eggs when you do not have enough left in your refrigerator or want to try an alternative. Eggs are a good source of protein, vitamin E, calcium, and omega 3 healthy fats.

Question: Can I include canned vegetables or fish in place of fresh or frozen, when these options are not available?

Answer: Choosing canned foods should generally be avoided, though when fresh and frozen are not available, canned can be chosen. It is important to determine which types of canned foods are best to include, as some are better than others. For example, vegetables tend to contain more sodium and preservatives in some cans, whereas others may be low in sodium and other ingredients. Canned fish is generally acceptable, and the best option for salmon and tuna is with water (not oil), as it can be easily drained and used without any preservatives. Canned fruits should generally be avoided because they are almost always packaged in a strong syrup that contains a high level of sugar and preservatives. Fish, tomato sauce (crushed or diced tomatoes), and select vegetables in cans are usually the best option for a balanced diet when you cannot find or source fresh or frozen foods. This can especially be challenging if you live in a northern climate during winter months. If you need to rely on canned foods that may contain preservatives, make sure you drink plenty of water and add other anti-inflammatory foods, balance your diet, and avoid the ill effects of preserved foods.

Question: Are some forms of inflammation an important sign or the body's way of fighting disease? If so, how do I know?

Answer: Inflammation will occur when you are infected with a virus or your body is fighting a disease, though it will often disappear once you have overcome it. Inflammation becomes problematic when it is recurring and painful. When this happens, your body is in a constant state of swelling and pain as a side effect of arthritis, fibromyalgia, and other similar chronic conditions that can have many long-term effects on the body. When this occurs, your body isn't fighting infection or disease, but constantly dealing with inflammation as a warning sign that other factors are causing distress and harm to the body. By reducing inflammation with a balanced diet and active lifestyle, you will notice an improvement in your health overall, including the conditions that may be triggering inflammation.

Question: Is it recommended to reduce red meat and dairy, or should I eliminate these foods?

Answer: Red meat and dairy can contribute to inflammation and high acidic levels in the body, though in moderation, and in combination with a diet heavy in plant-based foods, you can enjoy a pork roast or grilled cheese now and again. The key is balance, and making sure that you avoid too many acid-producing foods is kept to keeping the effects of inflammation reduced as much as possible. If you choose to follow a plant-based diet, this is an ideal plan and will prevent a lot of high acid foods, as the majority (if not all) plant-based foods are alkaline based and are easier for your body to digest.

Question: Should I use supplements for the nutrients not included in my diet?

Answer: A nutrient-rich diet is the best option for eating well. Supplements are a good option if you cannot receive all the vitamins and minerals required or live in a region where certain foods and/or nutrients are difficult to find. For example, vitamin D is often taken in supplement form as a tablet or drops in northern climates where sunlight is reduced, especially during colder months. Supplements are also important for people who are deficient in certain nutrients, such as iron, calcium, or protein. A multivitamin is a way that many people ensure they are getting everything they need daily just in case their meals and food choices do not include certain nutrients they may need.

Choosing a supplement is an important process that should involve research and consulting with a medical professional or dietician to ensure you find the right option for you.

Question: Are soy-based foods safe to include in my diet regularly?

Answer: Yes, soy-based food is an excellent food that is not only plant-based but high in alkaline while reducing or eliminating inflammation. There is a wealth of nutrients in soybeans, including their raw form, edamame beans, as well as tofu, miso, tempeh, and other forms of soy. Some people can experience soy-related food sensitivities and allergies, though some fermented versions of soy are easier to digest and enjoy when regular tofu or soy-based beverages are not suitable. Miso paste, soup, and tempeh are examples of fermented soy that can add a wealth of nutrients into your diet, including vitamin B12, calcium, protein, fiber, and many other vitamins and minerals. Soy is low in carbohydrates and doesn't contain trans fats, which makes it beneficial for weight loss, while getting all the protein and calcium you need, without animal-based foods.

Eating soy daily is safe, though it is important to choose good quality soy foods. If possible, focus on organic and locally grown varieties of soy, and avoid smoked or high sodium versions of tofu and tempeh, which can add artificial ingredients that can reverse the benefits of nutrients in these foods.

Question: Are there any restrictions for following the anti-inflammation diet, and how will this way of eating impact people with allergies and food sensitivities?

Answer: One of the greatest advantages of the anti-inflammation diet is the ability to pick and choose the foods you want to include, which can mean replacing certain ingredients and foods with other options, which also reduce inflammation. Many plant-based foods offer excellent alternatives to meat, soy, and foods that contain gluten. Jackfruit, lentils, beans, legumes, and coconut-based yogurts are excellent examples of foods that can easily readily be used in place of dairy and meat. The anti-inflammation diet allows for a lot of customizing in your meal planning, including the recipes included in this book, which are ideal for experimenting with a variety of flours, sweeteners, fruits, vegetables, and many other options.

Question: If I "cheat" on this diet by eating foods that cause inflammation even just on occasion, will there be a long-term effect?

Answer: Now and again, it is natural to take a break from your regular diet, which is acceptable in moderation. You may notice a greater effect on your body if you have successfully reduced or stopped inflammation completely. For example, an instance of inflammation may suddenly occur after a "cheat" meal or snack that can trigger it. You may feel more bloating or indigestion as well. If this happens, drink plenty of water and rest. A small serving of yogurt, ginger tea, or green tea can help settle the stomach and aid digestion. Avoid heavily processed and deep-fried foods as much as possible to minimize the negative impact of these foods.

Final Tips and Suggestions for a Successful Anti-inflammatory Diet

As you move towards eating a healthier, most sustainable diet for the long-term, it's important to keep a few suggestions and tips in mind to ensure your success. For many people, a dietary change is seen as temporary, though once they return to eating the same way in the past, they quickly notice a decline in health and inflammation will soon return. Keeping your health optimal and eating well requires effort, though it can be an enjoyable experience that doesn't have to be unpleasant or difficult. Once your body adjusts to eating better, you'll want to avoid all the unhealthy, processed foods commonly found in your local supermarket or food stores.

1. Don't feel rushed to change your diet all at once. You don't have to have to dump all the foods you currently eat for a new set of dietary rules suddenly. Taking this approach can hinder your success in the long term, as you discover that making too many drastic switches at once can cause your body to crave the unhealthy food options you wish to stop. For this reason, make gradual switches and reduce the amount of the unhealthy foods you want to eliminate. For example, switching from sugar to honey or maple syrup, or eating a bowl of fresh fruit or berries instead of ice cream are examples of simple, but useful changes that make a major impact on your diet early, without a complete overhaul. If your diet

needs an overhaul, do this gradually, too, so that you're not risking sliding back into the habit of eating unhealthy or inflammatory foods.

2. Stay focused and don't give up. If you view your diet journey as an "all or nothing" approach, it will only become more difficult when you make a mistake or "cheat" with a food that you would otherwise avoid. Make your progress count with small, meaningful changes that last, instead of feeling let down when you slide back a few steps. It's natural and normal to crave the foods you have enjoyed for years, and when you switch them for healthier choices, it can feel odd at first. Replacing certain foods and cutting down on others, little by little, is the best method for success, and can give you a better sense of satisfaction in the long-term (and the short-term too!)

3. Be wary of fad diets and trends. There are many good intentions and healthy diets to follow, though not every plan works equally for everyone. For example, a low carb diet is exceptional for certain people and can bring about quick and long-lasting results, whereas other people may find it does less for them, and may even increase certain health risks if they do not follow the diet correctly, or take shortcuts. If you decide to follow a diet for health and/or weight loss, ensure that you research the benefits and disadvantages thoroughly, and consult a doctor or medical

professional before you begin. Some diets work well with anti-inflammatory foods, while others may not, which is important to confirm and understand before you consider following any dietary plan.

4. You don't have to count calories or become fixated on carbohydrates. Not all carbs are the same, and counting calories can be not only discouraging but counterproductive. The key to eating well and keeping your health and weight within a reasonable level is with good quality, natural foods with little or no preservatives. For example, eating low carb foods isn't going to benefit your health if none of these foods are high in nutrients. If you rely on packaged foods to advertise or claim their nutritious value, you'll find they do not always live up to their standards, and cannot replicate the natural sources of vitamins and nutrients found in natural foods, such as fruits, vegetables, natural meats, fish, nuts, and seeds. Focus on quality, not quantity, and you'll find the results will not only be what you're looking for but last longer as well.

5. If you have friends or family interested in making positive dietary changes, it can be advantageous to make better food choices together, as well as shopping, cooking, baking, and sharing recipes. We are often more motivated when our peers and family want to give a new diet or food trend a try and following the anti-inflammatory diet is a great option for many people, as it focuses more on

food choices and health, and not as much on calories and carbohydrates.

6. The quality of food is of the utmost importance. This applies to all your food choices and the ingredients you choose for your recipes. Local, high quality, and, if possible, organic produce, meat, and dairy are ideal. Focus on whole foods as much as possible and avoid dried or canned foods unless this is the only option. If you choose a canned or dried good, make sure there is little or no preservatives, or additives. Canned foods can be rinsed and drained to minimize the effect of sodium and other ingredients used for preservation.

7. Expand your palate! Anti-inflammatory foods, which include a wide range of choices, and this means opening your mind to the possibility of trying new and interesting fruits and vegetables that you may never have considered before. There may be some imported fruit or even a locally grown vegetable that piques your interest, even if you're uncertain whether or not to try it. Some foods are excellent for texture and taste. If you're not sure whether a specific food or ingredient will taste good, try a small sample at first. You may be surprised at the result, and in some cases, develop a taste for something new and different!

Adapting to a new diet comes with many changes, and the anti-inflammation diet is no exception. There is a focus more on eating healthy and less on weight loss, though by following and adjusting your eating habits to reduce or eliminate inflammation you'll notice many other positive results as well.

Conclusion

As you begin following the anti-inflammation diet, you will notice some effects in the short-term, while the long-term results are excellent for many improvements that impact your health, such as lower risk in heart disease, cancer, and reducing the effects of chronic conditions. The anti-inflammation diet or way of eating provides many options that can be individually customized for any dietary plan, either due to allergies and food sensitivities or preferences. While the diet is highly plant-based, including moderate amounts of lean meats and seafood is a great balance and helps ensure that you get the type of benefit of healthy fats and protein. Through experimenting with the recipes in this book and following the general guidelines of following the anti-inflammation diet, you'll see a lot of progress in a short period. The key to success is consistency and focusing on your health. From this starting point, you'll notice many ...

If you enjoyed this book, please let me know your thoughts by leaving a short review on Amazon. Thank you

"Other books by Alexander Great"

Autoimmune Protocol Diet*: The Complete Guide to the Protocol to Improving Your Health With the Autoimmune Diet:*
https://www.amazon.com/dp/B08D2J6V37

Autoimmune Diet for Beginners*: Complete Step-By-Step Guide to Cooking Healthy Dishes and Losing Weight Quickly With the Autoimmune Diet:*
https://www.amazon.com/dp/B08D1VYW6F

Autoimmune Diet Cookbook*: Complete Step-By-Step Guide to Cooking Healthy Dishes and Increase Immune Defenses With The Autoimmune Solution:*
https://www.amazon.com/dp/B08D3Y66G7

AIP Diet : *4 Manuscripts: Autoimmune Protocol Diet Autoimmune Disease Anti-Inflammatory Diet, Autoimmune Diet for Beginners, Autoimmune Diet Cookbook*
https://www.amazon.com/dp/B08JWP59MD